The New Leadership Challenge

Creating the Future of Nursing

THIRD EDITION

The New Leadership Challenge

Creating the Future of Nursing

THIRD EDITION

Sheila C. Grossman, PhD, APRN-BC
Professor & Director of Family Nurse Practitioner Track
School of Nursing
Fairfield University
Fairfield, Connecticut

Theresa M. Valiga, EdD, RN, FAAN
Director, Institute for Educational Excellence
Duke University School of Nursing
Durham, North Carolina

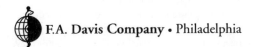 F.A. Davis Company • Philadelphia

F.A. Davis Company
1915 Arch Street
Philadelphia, PA 19103
www.fadavis.com

Copyright © 2009 by F.A. Davis Company.

Printed in the United States of America

Last digit indicates print number: 10 9 8 7 6 5 4

Publisher, Nursing: Joanne Patzek DaCunha, RN, MSN
Director of Content Development: Darlene D. Pedersen
Project Editor: Padraic J. Maroney
Design and Illustration Manager: Carolyn O'Brien

As new scientific information becomes available through basic and clinical research, recommended treatments and drug therapies undergo changes. The author(s) and publisher have done everything possible to make this book accurate, up to date, and in accord with accepted standards at the time of publication. The author(s), editors, and publisher are not responsible for errors or omissions or for consequences from application of the book, and make no warranty, expressed or implied, in regard to the contents of the book. Any practice described in this book should be applied by the reader in accordance with professional standards of care used in regard to the unique circumstances that may apply in each situation. The reader is advised always to check product information (package inserts) for changes and new information regarding dose and contraindications before administering any drug. Caution is especially urged when using new or infrequently ordered drugs.

Library of Congress Cataloging-in-Publication Data

Grossman, Sheila.
The new leadership challenge : creating the future of nursing/Sheila C. Grossman, Theresa M. Valiga. – 3rd ed.
    p. ; cm.
Includes bibliographical references and index.
ISBN-13: 978-0-8036-2045-2
ISBN-10: 0-8036-2045-4
1. Nurse administrators. 2. Leadership. I. Valiga, Theresa M. II. Title.
[DNLM: 1. Nursing, Supervisory. 2. Leadership. 3. Nurse Administrators. WY 105 G8785n 2009]
RT89.G77 2009
362.17'3068–dc22

2008009995

Dedication

This book is dedicated to each and every nurse who is leading the profession to a preferred future and to my students, patients, mentors, and colleagues who have taught me so much about staying committed to a vision of enhancing leadership and followership. Also, I want to thank my husband, Bob; our daughters, Lisa and Beth; and my parents, sister, and brother, who have always inspired me to keep on task and do my best.

SCG

This book is dedicated to the many faculty and other professional colleagues, as well as the hundreds of students I have known who have helped me crystallize my thinking about leadership and who, themselves, have taken on the challenge of providing leadership. Through dialogues in the classroom, papers that have been written, conversations in each other's offices, sharing of resources and ideas, and observing these individuals functioning as leaders, I have come to understand more fully the true meaning of what it means to be a leader. I also dedicate this book to my husband, Bob, who continues to support me in all my professional pursuits and whose patience and understanding have meant the world to me. This book also is dedicated to my sister, Diane Czerepuszko, a nurse, a leader, a friend. Finally, I dedicate this book to my mother and father. Although neither of them is here to see its publication, they were a tremendous influence in my development as a professional and, hopefully, a leader; for that and for all they have given me, I will be forever grateful.

TMV

Author Biographies

Sheila C. Grossman, PhD, APRN-BC, received her baccalaureate degree in nursing and her doctoral degree in higher education professional administration from the University of Connecticut, her master's degree from the University of Massachusetts in biophysiological nursing with a clinical nurse specialty in respiratory nursing, and her post masters certificate as a Family Nurse Practitioner from Fairfield University. Dr. Grossman has completed the Cincinnati Children's Hospital Genetics Fellowship and the AACN Leadership Fellowship. She has been a staff and charge nurse on a variety of medical-surgical units and intensive care units. She has been a critical care nursing instructor at Hartford Hospital and St. Francis Hospital and Medical Center, both in Hartford, CT. She has taught nursing at the University of Connecticut and currently is a Professor and Director, Family Nurse Practitioner Track in the School of Nursing at Fairfield University (CT), affiliating clinically at the Yale New Haven Hospital. She works as a nurse practitioner every week at Trinity Health Center in Hartford, CT. Dr. Grossman has done multiple national and local presentations and publications in the areas of pathophysiology, geriatrics, palliative care, primary care and critical care nursing outcome studies, mentoring, leadership, and evidence-based practice. She is a past member of the Connecticut State Board of Nursing and a member of Sigma Theta Tau International, American Association of Critical Care Nurses, and the American Academy of Nurse Practitioners.

Theresa M. Valiga, EdD, RN, FAAN, received her bachelor's degree in nursing from Trenton State College (now The College of New Jersey) and her master's and doctoral degrees, both in nursing education, from Teachers College, Columbia University. She has been a faculty member at Trenton State College, Georgetown University, Seton Hall University, Villanova University, and Fairfield University, where she served as Dean of the School of Nursing. At present, she is the Director of the newly created Institute for Educational Excellence in the School of Nursing at Duke University (N.C.). Prior to this position, Dr. Valiga served for 9 years as the Chief Program Officer at the National League for Nursing. Dr. Valiga's primary research interests relate to students' cognitive/intellectual development, critical thinking, and leadership development. Her publications, presentations, and consultations center around these topics, as well as curriculum development, creative teaching strategies, and various professional issues. She is the author of several articles and has coauthored two other books: *The Nurse Educator in Academe: Strategies for Success* and *Using the Arts and Humanities to Teach Nursing: A Creative Approach*. She has served as Vice President of Sigma Theta Tau International and National Vice President of the Interdisciplinary Honor Society of Phi Kappa Phi, and she has held numerous leadership positions in nursing throughout her career. Dr. Valiga also is the recipient of several awards, including the Sigma Theta Tau International Founders Award for Excellence in Education and the National League for Nursing Isabel Stewart Award for Excellence in Nursing Education, and she is a Fellow in the American Academy of Nursing.

Foreword

In my mind, the word leadership evokes the image of travel. I see a ship out front, leading the way, helping others move from point A to point B. When one leads the minds of others from one point to another, we call it education.

I have come to understand that education is a natural leadership opportunity. Some of our greatest leaders may have been those who have assisted in the framing and reframing of our minds. Education does not only happen in the halls of academe. There are equal opportunities for major and minor miracles to occur in the lived world of nursing practice.

It is from these two vantage points, that of the clinician and the educator, that the authors of this book, Drs. Sheila Grossman and Terry Valiga, share their collective and collected knowledge of leadership. They are clearly not interested in leadership for the sake of leadership. Rather, they have designed this book to co-create the future of nursing. With subtlety, they challenge all nurse leaders—in education, practice, administration, research, consultation, and any other role—to self-assess their own leadership capacity.

While this book is incredibly useful for teaching undergraduate and graduate nurses about leadership, it is also well positioned to revitalize the existing and old guard of leadership in nursing and focus our attention on the primary task of leading health care transformation. Nursing's future is intertwined with the future of health care. Nursing and patient care are two sides of the same coin. By revitalizing health care, we create the future of nursing.

This is a book of surprises. With grace and elegance, the authors present the concepts and realities of leadership, bringing together academic analysis and poetry in a way that is truly amazing. They foreshadow, for example, evidence-based information about leadership with voices as disparate as those of Kipling and Kennedy. Each chapter is a teacher's master plan, with learning objectives and critical thinking exercises. But the topics cover that which is difficult to grasp: visions, dreams, and chaos. Using this text will require the educator to engage with others (students, perhaps) in mutual discovery and inquiry. This approach does not draw conclusions but opens the way to dialogue, reflection, and exploration as part of the leadership journey.

This book is an essential tool for developing leaders and for maintaining one's own leadership ability, passion, and commitment. It inspires us to look at the stars, to envision possibilities, and begin to lead. It has the potential to demystify leadership and simultaneously maintain the spirit and magic of inspiration. Colleagues, I am honored to invite you to turn the page and begin your exploration of the subterranean structures of leadership and new pathways toward the future of health care and the future of nursing.

Beverly Malone, PhD, RN, FAAN
Chief Executive Officer
National League for Nursing

Preface

The New Leadership Challenge: Creating the Future of Nursing has been written as a reference book and textbook for undergraduate or graduate students in nursing, as well as for nurses in any practice role. The book also will be helpful for nurses pursuing graduate study, including those preparing as clinical nurse leaders or those pursuing a doctorate of nursing practice. It provides an overview of major ideas related to the multidimensional concept of "leadership" and explores those ideas at various levels of one's career development: beginning, intermediate, and advanced.

Each chapter includes learning objectives, a synthesis of extensive readings (from nursing, and more often, non-nursing literature) on the specific topic, a case study, and a variety of critical thinking exercises that are designed to help the reader better understand the topic and its relation to leadership and the development of individuals as leaders. Resources from the arts and humanities that relate to the specific topic and that enhance learning about it are provided, and examples from clinical practice, education, and administration are included.

Unlike many other textbooks and resource books that address leadership, this book takes that charge seriously. In many other books, particularly those written by and for nurses and nursing students, the authors confuse leadership with management and end up focusing more on management than on leadership. Perhaps that is because the phenomenon of leadership is more elusive than that of management and because one cannot outline "steps" of leadership as one can do to some extent with management (e.g., planning, delegating, budgeting).

This book takes on the challenge of exploring the elements of true leadership, particularly in the "new world" context we face continually. It explores various definitions and conceptualizations of leadership, examines extant theories of leadership, analyzes the notion of vision and visionary leadership, and tackles the intricacies of leader-follower relationships. The importance of followership, the facilitation of change, the management of conflict, the use and abuse of power, gender issues in leadership, and the development of oneself and of others as leaders all are discussed. In essence, then, this book takes a broad look at the complex phenomenon of leadership and examines multiple dimensions of it.

The major points made throughout this book and its unifying elements are as follows: (1) although leadership and management are related, they are not one and the same; (2) leadership is not an innate ability but one that can be learned and developed through conscious and purposeful effort; (3) each of us can be and, perhaps, needs to be a leader if nursing is to advance as a profession and have a significant impact in the twenty-first century; and (4) there are ways in which each of us can develop as a leader throughout our careers. These points are made and the goals of the book achieved through a balance of theoretical exploration; the extensive use of real-world examples from clinical practice, education, and administration; self-assessment exercises; and the integration of creative learning activities.

The New Leadership Challenge: Creating the Future of Nursing focuses on nurses and nursing. It does not confuse leadership and management. It also explores the multifaceted concept of leadership in depth. As such, it is of value to several audiences.

Most undergraduate programs include a course in nursing leadership. A study conducted by one of the authors and another colleague revealed, however, that although many courses carried the title "Nursing Leadership," most actually dealt with management and delegation. In a world where experts recognize clearly that true leadership is needed for the future, *The New Leadership Challenge: Creating the Future of Nursing* meets a need, particularly for those undergraduate programs that already have or will soon have a course that addresses true leadership.

Most graduate programs focus on the preparation of graduates for leadership roles in the profession, so a book that addresses just that is most appropriate. Students preparing as educators or nurse practitioners do not want to use a text that "advertises" leadership but "delivers" management; if they wanted management, they would have pursued an MBA or a graduate degree in nursing administration. Instead, they want a text that helps them understand what leadership is and how it relates to the roles for which they are preparing. This book meets that need.

Finally, this book serves as a valuable resource for nurses in clinical practice, nurse educators, and nurse administrators who see the need to learn more about the phenomenon of leadership and how to develop those abilities in themselves and in others (e.g., fellow clinicians, students, one's staff). One's ongoing education in an ever-changing world cannot be limited to clinical, teaching, or administrative knowledge and skills alone. It also must address broader knowledge and skills—such as those related to leadership—that are integral to one's practice.

One of the most important features of this book is the exposure to and integration of the extensive writings about leadership done by experts in that field; thus, the literature base for this book is not limited to nursing. This is designed to broaden the readers' perspectives and expose them to a much wider range of resources that can be tapped for ongoing personal development. The annotated summaries of "must-read" books on leadership included in this 3rd edition are intended to help readers expand their horizons about leadership resources.

The New Leadership Challenge: Creating the Future of Nursing, as the title implies, also presents a clear orientation to the future. Using the writings of Wheatley as a basis, the entire book is "framed" in the context of the future—what organizations are expected to look like in the future, the skills that people associated with those organizations will need to survive and thrive, the need to plan for a blending of professional and personal commitments, and so on. The old-model, hierarchic organization that characterizes so many healthcare agencies is expected to "die" very quickly, and people in those organizations will need to be able to function and provide leadership in a totally new kind of environment. This book is designed to help professional nurses make this transition.

In addition to these important features, *The New Leadership Challenge: Creating the Future of Nursing* offers several other unique features. First, it is accompanied by an instructor's guide that offers numerous teaching approaches that might be used with undergraduate or graduate students and with nurses in practice. Overall, this book—conceptualized in its broadest sense—is designed to be interactive, stimulating, creative, challenging, and thought-provoking.

The intent of this book is to help nurses and nursing students explore the many facets of leadership and examine strategies that will aid them in (1) seeing themselves as potential leaders, (2) developing skills needed to function as leaders, and (3) taking on the challenges of a leadership role in the current and future healthcare setting. It challenges the reader's thinking, presents new ways to conceptualize leadership, and prepares nurses for their role as leaders in creating a preferred future for nursing. Readers are invited to open their minds to new perspectives; entertain the notion that the chaotic, uncertain world of today and tomorrow presents tremendous opportunities for nurse leaders to influence the future of our profession; and think of themselves as leaders who can develop in that role throughout their careers. We welcome you to the world of *The New Leadership Challenge: Creating the Future of Nursing.*

Sheila C. Grossman
Theresa M. Valiga

Reviewers

Sonia Acorn PhD, RN
Professor Emerita
The University of British Columbia
Wesbrook Mall
Vancouver, British Columbia, Canada
Instructor
Athabasca University
Athabasca, Alberta Canada

William D. Ahrens MSN, RN
Instructor
University of North Florida
Jacksonville, Florida

Sandra Filice BAAN, MS
Program Coordinator
Humber College
Toronto, Ontario, Canada

Reynaldo Rivera MA, EdM, APRN, RN, CCRN, CNAA, BC
Director of Special Programs
New York Presbyterian Hospital, Weill Cornell Medical Center
New York, New York

Acknowledgments

The authors wish to thank Joanne DaCunha for inviting us to explore the concept of leadership through a textbook and for her innovative ideas about what this book could be. We will always be grateful for her inspiration, her faith in us, and her ongoing support with the project and the revised editions.

Our gratitude also is extended to Dr. Beverly Malone for her thoughtful reflections in the Foreword to this book. Finally, we thank our families and friends for their love and support throughout the process of developing and writing this book.

SCG
TMV

Contents

Chapter 1   **The Nature of Leadership: Distinguishing Leadership from Management**   **1**

Brief Overview of Selected Theories of Leadership   2
Leadership and Management   3
Tasks of Leadership   4
Specific Distinctions Between Leadership and Management   4
Elements of Leadership   7

Chapter 2   **The New World and New Leadership: Changing Our Thinking About Leadership**   **23**

Preparing Nurse Leaders   24
Chaos Theory   25
Quantum Theory and the New Science   27
Supporting Perspectives and Perspective Transformation Theory   29

Chapter 3   **Followership and Empowerment**   **35**

The Concept of Followership   39
Types of Followers   41
Characteristics of Effective or Exemplary Followers   44
Sources of Power   46
Empowering Self and Others   48
Strategies to Develop Effective Followership Skills   49

Chapter 4   **Leadership as an Integral Component of a Professional Role**   **61**

Types of Leadership   63
Emotional Intelligence   65

	Self-Esteem and Leadership Image	66
	Would-Be Leaders Become Leaders	67
	Leadership as an Integral Component of Each Nurse's Role	68
Chapter 5	**Vision and Creativity**	**75**
	The Concept of Vision	76
	Why Have a Vision?	77
	The Process of Creativity	85
Chapter 6	**Gender Perspectives in Leadership**	**99**
	Common Gender Differences	100
	Women's Ways of Leading	102
	Combining the Best of "Femaleness" and "Maleness"	106
	Strategies for Women and Men to be Successful Leaders in the Future	108
Chapter 7	**Disequilibrium and Chaos: Invigorating, Challenging, and Growth-Producing**	**115**
	Adjusting the Leader Role and the Practice of Leadership	116
	Defining of Chaos	117
	Chaos in Nursing	119
	Complexity of the Registered Nurse Role in the Current Healthcare System	120
	Facilitating Leadership in Chaos	121
	Change	122
	The Leader as a Change Agent	123
	Facilitating the Change Process	125
	The Process of Change	127
	Barriers to Change	128
	Dealing with Conflict Generated by Change	128
Chapter 8	**Shaping a Preferred Future for Nursing**	**137**
	Predicting the Future	138
	General Predictions About the Future	142
	Predictions About the Future of Healthcare	143
	Predictions About the Future of Nursing	145
	Characteristics of Nurse Leaders Needed to Create a Preferred Future for Nursing	151
Chapter 9	**Developing as a Leader Throughout One's Career**	**157**
	General Approaches to Leadership Development	158
	Environments That Facilitate Leadership Development	165
	Empowerment	167
	Mentoring	168
	Networking	172

Chapter 10   **Conclusion**   **181**
                  The Concept of Excellence   182
                  Leadership and Excellence   188
                  Professional Involvement   189

Annotated Bibliography   **195**
Index   **225**

CHAPTER 1

The Nature of Leadership:
Distinguishing Leadership from Management

> **LEARNING OBJECTIVES**
> - Compare and contrast major theoretical ideas about leadership.
> - Discuss the essential elements of leadership.
> - Describe the nine tasks of leadership.
> - Distinguish leadership from management.
> - Create a personal definition of leadership that reflects its essential elements.

INTRODUCTION

Chaos. Uncertainty. Unpredictability. Constant change. These are all characteristics of the world in which we now live, and all indications are that the world of the future will be even more chaotic, more uncertain, more unpredictable, and in even greater states of constant and unprecedented change and flux. Such circumstances desperately call for new leaders. Indeed, "if there was ever a moment in history when a comprehensive strategic view of leadership was needed, . . . this is certainly it" (Bennis & Nanus, 1985, p. 2).

Defining just what leadership is, who leaders are, what leaders do, and how leadership is different from management—a phenomenon with which it often is confused—is no easy task. This chapter is intended to address these questions and help the reader understand the complex, multidimensional concept we refer to as leadership. It is also intended to challenge readers to consider the leadership we need in nursing today, to think about themselves as leaders, and to reflect on how leadership responsibilities can be integrated into their roles as professional nurses.

For almost a century, writers have attempted to describe leadership, and researchers have attempted to identify the defining characteristics of leaders. The outcome has been one very clear conclusion: "Leadership is one of the most observed and least understood phenomena on earth" (Burns, 1978, p. 2). It is multidimensional and multifaceted—a universal human phenomenon that many know when they see it, but few can define clearly.

In fact, "there are almost as many different definitions of leadership as there are persons who have attempted to define the concept" (Bass, 1990). According to Bennis and Nanus (1985, p. 4): "Decades of academic analysis have given us more than 350 definitions of leadership. Literally thousands of empirical investigations of leaders have been conducted in the last seventy-five years alone, but no clear and unequivocal understanding exists as to what distinguishes leaders from non-leaders, and perhaps more important, what distinguishes *effective* leaders from *ineffective* leaders" (p. 11).

The lack of a "clear and unequivocal understanding" of leadership has led these experts on the subject to assert that "never have so many labored so long to say so little" (p. 4). Despite this situation, however, there is increasing clarity about what true leadership is and how it is different from the related concept of management.

BRIEF OVERVIEW OF SELECTED THEORIES OF LEADERSHIP
Great Man Theory

Theories of leadership have evolved tremendously over the years (Bass, 1990, pp. 37–55). Among the earliest was the "Great Man Theory," which asserted that one was a leader if one was born into the "right" family—usually a family of nobility—and possessed unique characteristics, most of which were inherited. Although some individuals who were born into the "right" family did accomplish extraordinary things and did, in fact, change the course of history, the notion that "leaders are born, not made" did not capture the imagination of the masses, and it failed to recognize that there was more to leadership than having royal blood. Thus began the search for the traits or cluster of traits that would determine whether a person would be a leader.

Trait Theories

Personal trait theories of leadership attempted to distinguish leaders from other people and identify the universal characteristics of leadership. Not surprisingly, no qualities were found that were universal to all leaders, although a number of traits did seem to correlate with leadership (Bass, 1990): above average height and weight, an abundant reserve of energy, an ability to maintain a high level of activity, better education, superior judgment, decisiveness, a breadth of knowledge, a high degree of verbal facility, good interpersonal skills, self-confidence, and creativity. In addition to the fact that these theories revealed no universal traits among leaders, they also failed to acknowledge the importance of the situation in which leadership occurred.

Situational Theories

Situational theories, in comparison, gave clear recognition to the significance of the environment and the particular situation as factors in the effectiveness of a leader. They asserted that the leader was the individual who was in a position to institute change when a situation was ready for change. In other words, the leader did not plan for a change, nor was the leader chosen by a group of followers; he or she just "happened to be in the right place at the right time" and took the action that was needed to resolve a crisis or manage a problem. Although this view of leadership was broader than merely looking at one's heritage or specific traits, it still did not capture the complexity of the phenomenon and failed to acknowledge one very important element in a leadership "event"—the followers.

Contemporary Theories

More contemporary theories of leadership clearly recognize that effective leadership depends partly on the person of the leader, partly on the situation at hand, and partly on the qualities and maturity of the followers. In fact, most recent writings (Bennis, 2004; Burns, 2003; Chaleff, 1995; Collins, 2001; Corona, 1986; DePree, 1992; DiRienzo, 1994; Kelley, 1992, 1993; Lee, 1993; Pickens, 2000) assert that without followers, there is no leadership; followers therefore are a most significant element in the leadership "equation." Their needs, goals, abilities, sense of responsibility, degree of involvement, potentials, and so forth are all important in determining the effectiveness of a leader. In addition to acknowledging the significance of followers, more modern theories recognize that leadership is not a random occurrence. Instead, it very much involves having a vision, communicating that vision to others, planning with followers on how to make the vision a reality, effecting change, managing conflict, empowering followers, serving as a symbol for the group, serving as a source of energy and renewal for the group, and taking responsibility for facilitating the ongoing development of followers.

Leadership is, indeed, a complex, multifaceted phenomenon that does not "just happen" and is not limited to an elite few. It can be learned. It is deliberative. It is not necessarily tied to a position of authority. A leadership role is something each one of us has the potential to fulfill.

LEADERSHIP AND MANAGEMENT

The vast array of textbooks on leadership—particularly in nursing—often are titled "leadership and management." A careful analysis of the content of those textbooks often reveals, however, that a great deal of attention is given to management and very little to leadership. In fact, although the authors of many such textbooks make a point at the outset that leadership and management are not the same thing, they often go on to use the terms interchangeably and imply that the only person who is providing leadership to a group is the person who is in the management position. Nothing can be farther from the truth.

Although leadership and management are related and many managers are also leaders, these phenomena are not the same and should not be confused. Most important, one must remember that **leadership is not necessarily tied to a position of authority** and that each of us has the potential, and perhaps the responsibility, to provide leadership in our specific area of practice, our institution, our professional organizations, our community, and our profession as a whole.

TASKS OF LEADERSHIP

One of the most noted experts in the field of leadership, John Gardner, outlined nine tasks of leadership that help distinguish it from management. Those tasks of leadership (Gardner, 1989) are as follows:

1. *Envisioning goals:* Pointing others in the right direction and helping the group members balance and deal with any tension between long- and short-term goals
2. *Affirming values:* Regenerating and revitalizing the beliefs, values, purposes, and vision shared by members of the group, and challenging the values held by some
3. *Motivating:* Unlocking or channeling motives that exist within members of the group, having and promoting positive attitudes, being creative, and encouraging others to be excited about the future and about how they can be a part of it
4. *Managing:* Planning, setting priorities, making decisions, facilitating change, and keeping the system functioning, all in an effort to move the group toward achieving the goals and realizing the vision
5. *Achieving a workable unity:* Establishing trust, striving toward cohesion and mutual tolerance, managing conflict, and "creating loyalty to the larger venture" (p. 29)
6. *Explaining:* Helping others understand what the vision is, why they are being asked to do certain things, and how they relate to the larger picture
7. *Serving as a symbol:* Serving as a risk taker and acting as the group's source of unity, voice of anger, collective identity, and continuity, as well as its source of hope
8. *Representing the group:* Speaking and acting for or on behalf of the group and being an advocate for the group
9. *Renewing:* Blending continuity and change and breaking routines, habits, fixed attitudes, perceptions, assumptions, and unwritten rules

Gardner (1989) asserted that the *"sine qua non* of leadership" (p. 29) is the ability to achieve a workable unity in the group and build community. He also noted that in the process of renewing, the leader must "keep a measure of diversity and dissent in the system [as a way to avoid] the trance of nonrenewal" (p. 33). In essence, "leadership is not tidy" (p. 33); it is more of an art than a science. Management, in comparison, often is thought of as a science in which a series of steps can be followed to implement the role. Elements of the tasks of leadership will be explored in greater depth, but a careful look at how leadership differs from management can facilitate a more thorough understanding of leadership.

SPECIFIC DISTINCTIONS BETWEEN LEADERSHIP AND MANAGEMENT

Abraham Zaleznik (1981) has written extensively about the differences between leadership and management. In his classic work, Zaleznik asserted that leaders and managers are very different kinds of people: they differ in their motivation, their personal history, and how they think and act; they differ in their orientation toward goals, work, human relationships, and themselves; and they differ in their worldviews.

Goals

Leaders are proactive in formulating goals, primarily because they typically arise out of some personal passion for a better world. The goals are developed through dialogue with others, engagement with the literature, and self-reflection. Leaders shape ideas instead of merely responding to the ideas of others. They act to change the way people think about what is desirable, possible, and necessary. Managers, by comparison, adopt impersonal attitudes toward goals because someone higher in the organizational hierarchy often formulates those goals, which are deeply embedded in the history and culture of the organization, and arise out of necessity rather than passion and desire.

Conceptions of Work

Regarding their conceptions of work, leaders act to develop fresh approaches to long-standing problems and to open issues for new options. They are not satisfied with the status quo and tend to create an excitement in their work. Their instinct is to take risks, challenge "sacred cows," challenge existing assumptions, and ask "Why not?" Managers see work as a task to be accomplished with the least amount of turmoil and the greatest amount of coordination and balance. They act to limit choices and "rock the boat" as little as possible. Their instinct, in contrast to that of leaders, is for survival.

> *The cautious seldom err.* —Confucius

Relationships with Others

In their relationships with others, leaders are concerned with what events and decisions mean to those who are affected by them. They care about the people with whom they work, and they want to promote the development and individual creativity of their followers. They facilitate, focus on personal issues, and encourage the growth of others. Relationships with leaders may appear turbulent, intense, and, at times, even disorganized because of the involvement of all concerned. Despite this ability to work effectively with others, leaders are comfortable with solitary activity because it provides time for reflection, creative thinking, and incubation of ideas. Although managers are often thought of as "human engineers" (Holle & Blatchley, 1987) and like working with people, they tend to maintain a lower level of emotional involvement in their relationships with employees. They assign, focus on personnel issues, and promote the growth of the organization. They prefer to reconcile differences, seek compromises, and not become involved with what events mean to others. Instead, managers are concerned with how events occur, how things get done, and whether tasks are accomplished, preferably in the most efficient, cost-effective manner.

Sense of Self

Managers and leaders also have a different sense of self, according to Zaleznik (1981). Using the terms coined by William James many years ago, Zaleznik says leaders are "twice born" individuals—those who are separate from their environment, never "belong" to organizations, and have had many challenges in life. They are not threatened by the ideas of others because their sense of self comes from within, not from their roles or the expectations of others. Managers, on the other hand, often define themselves in terms of the organization and prefer not to have their ideas challenged. According to Zaleznik, they are "once born" individuals, whose lives are rather harmonious and who are very much influenced by others' opinions.

Table 1–1 summarizes these and other differences between leaders and managers. It is important to note that this table compares the extreme "ideal" leader with the extremely "organization-focused" manager for purposes of illustration. Although it may be difficult to do, many managers also serve as leaders in their organizations, and people in positions of authority are often leaders; therefore the distinctions are not as clear-cut as Table 1–1 may suggest. In fact, a recent analysis (Jennings, Scalzi, Rodgers, & Keane, 2007) suggests that today's healthcare environment requires managers/administrators to be leaders; therefore, the distinctions between these two roles are becoming increasingly blurred.

TABLE 1-1 Differences Between Leadership and Management		
	LEADERSHIP	MANAGEMENT
Position	Selected or allowed by a group of followers.	Appointed by someone higher in the organizational hierarchy.
Power Base	Comes from knowledge, credibility, and ability to motivate followers.	Arises from one's position of authority.
Goals/Visions	Arises from personal interests and passion that may not be synonymous with the goals of the organization.	Espoused or prescribed by the organization.
Innovative Ideas	Developed, tested, and encouraged among all members of the group.	Allowed, provided they do not interfere with task accomplishment, but not necessarily encouraged.
Risk Level	High risk, creativity, innovation.	Low risk, balance, maintaining the status quo.
Degree of Order	Relative disorder seems to be generated.	Rationality and control prevail.
Nature of Activities	Related to vision and judgment.	Related to efficiency and cost-effectiveness.
Focus	People.	Systems and structure.
Perspective	Long-range , with an eye on the horizon.	Short-range, with an eye on the bottom line.
Degree of "Freedom"	Freestanding and not limited to an organizational position of authority.	Tied to a designated position in an organization.
Actions	Does the right thing (Bennis & Nanus, 1985, p. 21).	Does things right (Bennis & Nanus, 1985, p. 21).

An important point to emphasize, however, is that **one can be a leader without being in a position of authority**. It is this aspect that professional nurses need to keep in mind when they face challenges in the practice arena: each one of us has the potential to provide leadership that will create new futures, and we need not be in a hierarchical position of authority to do that. In fact, if one considers how leaders "rock the boat," challenge existing ways of doing things, constantly ask "Why not?" questions, and are comfortable with—and indeed, thrive on—turmoil, one can see that it sometimes is easier to be a leader if one is *not* in a hierarchical position of authority.

> *Managers are people who do things right. Leaders are people who do the right thing.* —Warren Bennis & Burt Nanus

ELEMENTS OF LEADERSHIP

As noted, leadership is a complex, multifaceted phenomenon that has been defined in hundreds of ways. Despite these myriad definitions, however, several fundamental elements of leadership recur in writings about the concept. Those elements—vision, communication skills, change, stewardship, and developing and renewing followers (see Box 1–1)—are discussed in depth to help the reader gain a better understanding of leadership.

BOX 1-1 **Elements of Leadership**
Vision
Communication Skills
Change
Stewardship
Developing and Renewing Followers

Vision

Few would argue that having, creating, and expressing a vision is an important element of leadership. Manfredi (1995) asserted that one of the primary roles of leaders is that of creating visions—"engag[ing] in the process of traveling into the future" (p. 62). Leadership involves dreaming of possibilities, believing that there can be a better world, exploring uncharted waters, and asking questions such as "Why not?" Indeed, "great leaders create dreams that galvanize people into action" (Yeh, 2005, p. 13).

> *Leaders can conceive and articulate goals that lift people out of their petty preoccupations, carry them above the conflicts that tear a society apart, and unite them in a pursuit of objectives worthy of their best efforts.* —John Gardner

The significance of vision to leadership has been identified by numerous experts in the field (Bennis, 1989, 2004; DePree, 1989; Gardner, 1990; Hesselbein, Goldsmith, & Somerville, 1999; Jackman, 2005; Kouses & Posner, 1995; Nanus, 1992; Phillips, 1997; Thornberry, 2006). In fact, the ability to see a new world, or a different world, and mobilize others to help make it a reality is one of the hallmarks of leadership. Consider the following examples of individuals and their dreams, many of which became realities as a result of the individual's determination, persistence, and passion:

- **Henry Ford:** Affordable cars for "common" people
- **Mahatma Gandhi:** Freedom of the people of India
- **Steve Jobs:** Desktop computers for personal use
- **Martin Luther King, Jr.:** Racial equality
- **Candy Lightner:** Reduced drunk driving fatalities
- **Mother Teresa:** Compassionate care for the poorest of the poor
- **Florence Nightingale:** Reduced battlefield fatalities resulting from poor care
- **Robert Pittman:** A "marriage" between rock music and television
- **Fred Smith:** Overnight mail and package delivery, 365 days of the year
- **Sam Walton:** Affordable shopping in a family-oriented store

Cautious, careful people always casting about to preserve their reputation and social standing, never can bring about a reform. Those who are really in earnest must be willing to be anything or nothing in the world's estimation. —Susan B. Anthony

Although we think of these individuals today as major figures in our nation's or world's history, they were little-known men and women when their visions began to take shape, when they began talking to others about their vision, and when they initiated actions to turn those dreams into reality. As a result, we now see most people owning cars; the worldwide impact of the Sisters of Charity; greater racial equality; the effectiveness of Mothers Against Drunk Driving (MADD); the positive outcomes of nonviolence; freedom of people in various parts of the world; the success of Wal-Mart and Federal Express; a computer in many homes and offices; the impact of Music Television (MTV) on our nation's youth; and more scientific and nursing-oriented approaches to healtcare. It has been said that "in creating a vision, we are creating a power, not a place, an influence, not a destination" (Wheatley, 1999, p. 55). Surely, individuals like these have created a power and an influence that have touched millions.

As professional nurses in practice, each of us envisions a better world. We might think of ways to promote greater involvement of patients' families in care decisions or a more powerful role for the professional nurse on the healthcare team. We might see a more effective way to prepare patients for the transition from the critical care unit to a step-down unit or from the hospital to home care. We may look at ways to increase hospital stays for certain patients, such as those undergoing mastectomy, or encourage greater autonomy for the nurse in making referrals to needed services.

Whatever the vision, if it is something about which we care, as leaders, we cannot sit idle waiting for others to "make it happen." Instead, we must "think outside the box and . . . imagine all the places [we] can go" (Sturman, 2002, p. 36). As leaders, we must talk about our vision to other nurses, our nurse managers and administrators, patients, patients' families, other health professionals, members of the media, legislators—in fact, anyone who will or should listen. We must be passionate about the "little corner of the world" that needs change and take every opportunity to do something to make that change happen. We must move beyond "the walls of current policy, practice, procedure, and assumptions [as well as] the walls of the past—safe, familiar, and secure" (Hesselbein et al., 1999, p. 2). We do not have to be in positions of authority to raise the issues, to argue the necessity for the change, to elicit support for the idea, to speak eloquently and enthusiastically about possible solutions, or to convince others that it is a vision worth working toward. But we must have the vision.

> *The secret of leadership is . . . enthusiasm: winning others to your ideas by the joy you yourself feel in them.* —*J. Donald Walters*

Communication Skills

As can be seen from the preceding discussion and from a review of Gardner's (1989) tasks of leadership, leadership involves communicating one's ideas and visions, explaining to others (e.g., followers, group members) how that vision has relevance for them and how they can be a part of making it a reality, and inspiring others to invest their energies on behalf of the group and the goal. In essence, excellent communication skills are essential for effective leadership.

Individuals who have great ideas but refuse to share them with others or who communicate them in a way that does not generate excitement in others are not likely to see their visions become reality. Individuals who cannot help others clearly see the vision probably will not be very effective in convincing those potential followers to "join in the struggle." Likewise, individuals who are unable to listen to the ideas of others, respond to their suggestions, and convey an enthusiasm for input from all group members are not likely to be able to facilitate change, sustain an effort over time, or effectively manage the conflict that is almost certain to arise as new goals are being realized.

Nurses excel in communication. They know how to listen and how to encourage people to keep trying when there seems to be no hope of success or when the effort is extraordinarily difficult. They know how to encourage others to respond openly and how to overcome barriers to communication. Nurses are, therefore, particularly advantaged in this element of leadership, and they should use this skill to its fullest.

The public puts a great deal of trust in nurses, and the credibility of nurses is strong in the eyes of patients, families, legislators, and the general public. Nurses who provide leadership can benefit from this favorable perception by communicating their vision at every opportunity. Such opportunities are, in fact, more readily available than many nurses realize: serving on a committee at one's institution or professional association, speaking at a conference, writing for a professional journal or a local newspaper or organizational newsletter, meeting with a legislator, talking with patients and their families, being interviewed on a local radio station, holding office in one's professional association, campaigning for a candidate or a particular issue, confronting a healthcare team member, networking at professional meetings, forming alliances with other healthcare professionals, seeking and using a mentor, and so on. We are limited only by our imaginations and willingness to take risks.

Change

If leadership involves articulating and realizing visions, the process by which that happens is change. Indeed, "learning to lead is, on one level, learning to manage change" (Bennis, 1989, p. 145). Leaders, therefore, need to be effective change agents, knowing when change is needed, "stretch[ing] the imagination of followers" (Manfredi, 1995, p. 63) to appreciate the need for change, planning effectively for change to occur, involving those who will be affected by change in the process, helping others realize their role in making change and creating new worlds, maintaining a positive attitude throughout the challenges of change, and knowing when to maintain the status quo.

As Gardner (1990) noted, "leaders must understand the interweaving of continuity and change" (p. 124). They must realize that not all change is good or necessary and that changing only for the sake of changing is not always healthy. Therefore, continuity often is what a group needs, at least for a certain period. But leadership also involves a willingness to create change and manage the chaos that often is associated with change. It involves a willingness to embrace uncertainty (Clampitt & Dekoch, 2001) and risk failure rather than waiting for "guaranteed" success, and it involves keeping focused on the goal or vision.

Professional nurses have a responsibility to create change in their work or professional arenas. Nurses who are dissatisfied with the intake form used for new patients, for example, thinking it is not complete enough to provide an adequate database to plan long-term home care, can complain about the form to their colleagues and "blame" someone else for its inadequacies. But the professional nurse who is a leader will do more than just complain. He or she will outline what is needed to make the form complete, perhaps test it out in practice (by informally adapting the existing form), develop a plan for pilot testing on a wider scale, and propose how the new form could be integrated into the admission standards for nurses in that agency. Such an approach creates change that is intended to improve the overall quality of patient care, and although it takes more effort than merely complaining about the inadequacies of the existing intake form, the outcomes are worth the effort. As previously mentioned, leaders do not need to be in positions of authority, and they do not need to wait for "guaranteed" success before trying new approaches and creating change.

Leadership is action, not position. —Donald H. McGannon

Stewardship

"Stewardship is to hold something in trust for another" (Block, 1993, p. xx) and being responsible for something more than just oneself. It has to do with serving others, rather than serving our own self-interests or attempting to control others, and it involves a balance of power. In essence, stewardship incorporates "engendering partnerships" (Block, 1993, p. 6) and empowerment, and it occurs when one leads "with soul" (Bolman & Deal, 2001).

Block (1993) titled his first chapter "Replacing Leadership with Stewardship" and described leadership as "inevitably associated with behaviors of control, direction, and knowing what is best for others" (p. 13), noting that it "does not leave much room for the concept of partnership" (p. 17). Based on the previous discussion, Block's definition may be an appropriate one for management, but it is not at all consistent with leadership as it has been described here. Leadership and stewardship, therefore, are not necessarily opposites or incompatible phenomena. In fact, Block's discussion of stewardship as "creating something we care about so we can endure the sacrifice, risk, and adventure that commitment entails" (p. 10) is congruent with the elements of leadership described previously: deep commitment, risk taking, high energy, working with others, and an enormous investment of self.

If leaders are to move forward with creating new worlds and helping visions become realities, they must have a sense of stewardship. They must feel responsible for the "larger picture," oversee the implementation of change, ensure that it is the overarching vision that drives decisions and actions, establish partnerships with followers or group members, and give their personal self-interests a "back seat." They must, in the words of Robert Greenleaf (1977), be servant-leaders, those who "first serve others [and] whose primary motivation is a desire to help others" (Spears, 1995, p. 3).

Professional nurses at all levels need to have a sense of stewardship about their practice arenas—whether in the clinical area, education, administration, or research—and be concerned with overall excellence in those arenas. Educators, for example, who have a vision of creating positive learning experiences for students—where they are fully engaged in the learning process, work collaboratively with each other, are excited about what they are learning, use their creative and other potentials to the fullest, and use the teacher as a guide and a resource to facilitate their own learning—cannot be concerned with doing this only in their own courses. If they are to be leaders and demonstrate the essential element of stewardship, there must be an effort to see that such positive learning experiences are provided for students throughout the curriculum and a willingness to oversee that what is being done in the name of "positive learning experiences" is based on theory and research.

Developing and Renewing Followers

Finally, leadership involves the continual development of followers and ongoing renewal of their commitment, understanding, and involvement. In fact, Tichy (1997) asserted that one of the truly defining characteristics of leaders is their investment in creating leaders all around them.

More than accomplishing tasks or meeting deadlines, "leadership is about taking people to places where they have never dared to go . . . and building into the future by developing the abilities of others" (Tichy, 1997, p. xiv). Leaders who have a vision for the future need to ensure that there are people to carry that vision forward and continue to work to make it become a reality. Building toward a vision requires collaboration between leaders and followers, as well as a cadre of effective followers who provide leadership.

It is the leader's responsibility to build such a cadre and develop the next generation of leaders. Because "all people have untapped leadership potential" (Tichy, 1997, p. 6), part of the leader's role is to recognize that potential and capitalize on it so that an effort or change can be sustained. Developing and renewing others can occur through personal attention, role modeling, precepting, and mentoring, each of which is described briefly to show their similarities and differences.

Personal Attention
Personal attention involves the personal guidance one gives to another. It requires that the strengths, limitations, and goals of the "recipients" are known and are used as a basis for the challenges presented to those individuals, the opportunities made available to them, and the expectations that are set regarding their contributions to the group.

Role Modeling
Role modeling occurs when a more experienced individual performs a role in such a way that novice leaders follow the individual's actions, style, values, behaviors, and so on. Because one can be a role model for another without even knowing it, this method of developing and renewing others is considered a more passive approach.

Precepting
Precepting is a strategy often used in nursing in which an experienced individual may be "assigned" to teach, guide, and assist another who is learning a role. The preceptor relationship often has a specific time limitation, and specific responsibilities of the preceptor and preceptee are clearly outlined.

Mentoring
Mentoring, in comparison, is a purposeful relationship in which an experienced, accomplished individual chooses to enter into a relationship with a less experienced individual who shares certain values or goals, is seen as having potential, shares a certain "chemistry" with the mentor, and is willing to work with the mentor. Mentors "open doors" for protégés, give critical feedback and personal guidance about career goals and other significant matters, and are willing to enter into a relationship that may last for many years. When true mentoring occurs, protégés may accomplish professional goals that far exceed those of the mentor.

It is clear that there are many approaches to developing and renewing followers. Some are conscious and purposeful (e.g., mentoring, personal attention), some are "assigned" (e.g., precepting), and some may occur without the leader even being aware of their occurrence (e.g., role modeling). Regardless of the strategy used, the leader is committed to the development of the followers and to their continued renewal and involvement.

CONCLUSION

Leadership is a complex, multifaceted phenomenon that is quite different from management. It is a potential that each of us has, and a set of skills that can be learned, developed, and nurtured. Most important, it is not necessarily tied to a position of authority in an organization.

Opportunities exist in all aspects of our lives to exercise leadership and to make a difference in the lives of others and in the directions of groups and organizations. Leaders do not need to be appointed or even "invited" to exercise leadership; they do it because they "care more than others think is wise; risk more than others think is safe; dream more than others think is practical; and expect more than others think is possible" (anonymous quote about attaining excellence).

Never, never, never quit. —*Winston Churchill*

Leadership is needed for growth and progress—of individuals, groups, organizations, and institutions. As Harry Truman once said, "In periods where there is no leadership, society stands still. Progress occurs when courageous, skillful leaders seize the opportunity to change things for the better." In this world of increasing chaos, uncertainty, unpredictability, interdependence, and constant change, leadership is desperately needed. Nowhere is this more evident than in today's healthcare arena.

Professional nurses are in an excellent position to provide leadership within their work settings, professional associations, communities, and society at large. Their communication skills, ability to work collaboratively with others, sense of service to others, well-established credibility, and commitment to high-qualitypatient care make them excellent candidates to provide this much-needed leadership.

CRITICAL THINKING EXERCISES

Given the opportunity to publish "the definitive definition of leadership," what would you write? How does your definition reflect the nine tasks of leadership and the essential elements of leadership?

_____

_____

_____

Ask several nursing colleagues and several people outside the health professions (including children) to define leadership. What are the similarities in the definitions offered by these individuals? Are there any significant differences in their definitions? If so, what are they? How do you explain those differences?

_____

_____

If an alien came to earth, approached you, and said, "I see you are a nurse. Take me to your leader," to whom would you take the alien? Who, in your opinion, is providing true leadership within the profession or even within your own institution? Why would you take the alien to this person?

_____

_____

Read *The Velveteen Rabbit* (Williams, 1975). What leadership concepts can you identify in this children's story? What can we learn about leadership from this story?

_____

_____

Read the poem "If" by Rudyard Kipling. How do you think this relates to leadership and to the art of becoming a leader?

If

If you can keep your head when all about you
Are losing theirs and blaming it on you;
If you can trust yourself when all men doubt you
Yet make allowance for their doubting, too;
If you can wait and not be tired of waiting,

Continued

Or being lied about, don't deal in lies.
Or being hated, don't give way to hating,
And yet not look too good nor talk too wise;
If you can dream and not make dreams your master;
If you can think and not make thoughts your aim;
If you can meet with triumphs and disaster
And treat those two impostors just the same;
If you can bear to hear the truths you've spoken
Twisted by knaves to make a trap for fools,
Or see the things you gave your life to, broken
And stoop to build them up with worn-out tools;
If you can make one heap of all your winnings
And risk it on one turn of pitch and toss,
And lose and start again at your beginnings
And never breathe a word about your loss;
If you can force your heart and nerve and sinew
To serve your turn long after they are gone,
And so hold on when there's nothing in you
Except the will that says to them "hold on;"
If you can talk with crowds and keep your virtue,
Or walk with kings nor lose the common touch;
If neither foes nor loving friends can hurt you;
If all men count with you but none too much,
If you can fill the unforgiving minute
With sixty seconds worth of distance run—
Yours is the world and everything that's in it,
And—which is more—you'll be a man, my son!
—*Rudyard Kipling*

_____

_____

Complete the following two self-assessment tools to get a sense of how you "measure up" as a leader: (1) the "Grossman & Valiga Leadership Characteristics and Skills Assessment" tool, and (2) the "Leadership Skills: Rate Yourself" tool. How did you score? Were your scores consistent with how you think of yourself as a leader? Where were your greatest areas of strength?

_____

_____

THE GROSSMAN & VALIGA LEADERSHIP CHARACTERISTICS AND SKILLS ASSESSMENT

Directions: Part 1 lists statements that are useful in determining a person's perception of what makes a good leader. **Part 2** lists skills that are useful in determining a person's ability to lead. Answer "SA" to those statements with which you Strongly Agree and "A" to those statements with which you Agree. Answer "D" to those statements with which you Disagree and "SD" to those statements with which you Strongly Disagree.

	Part 1				
	STATEMENT	SA	A	D	SD
1	Leaders are very creative.				
2	The most important goal of a leader is to be sure the job gets done.				
3	Leaders should focus on people, not on the system.				
4	One does not need to be in a position of authority to be a leader.				
5	Credibility is an important characteristic of a leader.				
6	Leaders tend to be people with high energy who are passionate about their work.				
7	Leaders focus more on being creative than on accomplishing their vision or goal(s).				
8	Persistence is a trademark of an effective leader.				
9	Leaders are committed to their vision and tend not to adapt to change well.				
10	Leaders are good at empowering others to grow.				
11	It is important for leaders to have a dream and to be future-oriented.				
12	A person's ability to lead in a professional setting depends on his or her self-esteem.				
13	A leader's style of leading is determined by the situation and/or task at hand.				
14	A good leader must have integrity.				
15	Leaders mentor others to assist them in pursuing their dreams.				
16	Leadership is a quality one is born with, and it cannot be acquired.				
17	Good leaders help others to resolve conflict.				
18	One does not need to be an excellent critical thinker in order to be a great leader.				
19	A good leader should have excellent communication skills.				
20	Leaders always follow the rules.				

	Part 2				
	STATEMENT	SA	A	D	SD
1	I value integrity higher than power.				
2	People tend to think I have the ability to influence others.				
3	I feel confident about my knowledge base and skills, given my years of experience.				
4	I have a definite dream for where I want to be in my profession.				
5	I have mentored another person and found the experience rewarding.				
6	Change usually makes me feel nervous, and I tend to lose my self-confidence.				
7	I feel energized taking risks unless they are life threatening.				
8	I do not feel confident calling a physician about my patient's status.				
9	When I experience conflict, I usually give in and accommodate the other person.				
10	I feel I do make a difference as a nurse and plan to continue to do so.				
11	Since I am only a nurse, I am not responsible for patient care errors.				
12	I often follow others when I am not sure what to do about something.				
13	I notice I agree with others easily unless the issue is very dear to my heart.				
14	I attempt to empower ancillary workers because I find the team spirit is enhanced.				
15	Personally, I do not really have a vision as to where I plan to be in a few years.				
16	I enjoy conflict and rarely compromise my needs.				
17	I am an autonomous person.				
18	I have been told I am extremely reliable and dependable.				
19	I have great passion for my nursing career.				
20	It is important to me to think about and plan for the future.				

Scoring. Assign the number shown in the box below to the response you gave to each question **in Part 1** and each question in **Part 2.**

	Part 1			
	STATEMENT	SA	A	D	SD
1	Leaders are very creative.	4	3	0	0
2	The most important goal of a leader is to be sure the job gets done.	4	3	2	1
3	Leaders should focus on people, not on the system.	4	3	2	1
4	One does not need to be in a position of authority to be a leader.	4	3	0	0
5	Credibility is an important characteristic of a leader.	4	3	0	0
6	Leaders tend to be people with high energy who are passionate about their work.	4	3	0	0
7	Leaders focus more on being creative than on accomplishing their vision or goal(s).	4	3	3	4
8	Persistence is a trademark of an effective leader.	1	2	3	4
9	Leaders are committed to their vision and tend not to adapt to change well.	0	0	3	4
10	Leaders are good at empowering others to grow.	4	3	0	0
11	It is important for leaders to have a dream and to be future oriented.	4	3	0	0
12	A person's ability to lead in a professional setting depends on his or her self-esteem.	4	3	0	0
13	A leader's style of leading is determined by the situation and/or task at hand.	4	3	0	4
14	A good leader must have integrity.	4	3	2	1
15	Leaders mentor others to assist them in pursuing their dreams.	4	3	0	0
16	Leadership is a quality one is born with, and it cannot be acquired.	0	0	3	4
17	Good leaders help others to resolve conflict.	4	3	2	1
18	One does not need to be an excellent critical thinker in order to be a great leader.	0	0	3	4
19	A good leader should have excellent communication skills.	4	3	0	0
20	Leaders always follow the rules.	0	0	3	4

Interpretation of Scores

Part 1: Perception of what makes a good leader

Add up your score for Part 1. Here's what the scores indicate:

70 to 80 = Excellent perception of a good leader.

60 to 69 = Good perception of a good leader.

50 to 59 = Probably mixing up the difference between management and leadership.

40 to 49 = Definitely mixing up the difference between management and leadership.

39 or less = Need to do some reading on what good leadership is.

	STATEMENT	SA	A	D	SD
	Part 2				
1	I value integrity higher than power.	**4**	**3**	**0**	**0**
2	People tend to think I have the ability to influence others.	4	3	0	0
3	I feel confident about my knowledge base and skills, given my years of experience.	4	3	0	0
4	I have a definite dream for where I want to be in my profession.	4	3	3	4
5	I have mentored another person and found the experience rewarding.	4	3	0	0
6	Change usually makes me feel nervous, and I tend to lose my self-confidence.	4	3	0	0
7	I feel energized taking risks unless they are life threatening.	4	3	0	0
8	I do not feel confident calling a physician about my patient's status.	0	0	3	4
9	When I experience conflict, I usually give in and accommodate the other person.	0	0	3	4
10	I feel I do make a difference as a nurse and plan to continue to do so.	4	3	0	0
11	Since I am only a nurse, I am not responsible for patient care errors.	0	0	3	4
12	I often follow others when I am not sure what to do about something.	0	0	3	4
13	I notice I agree with others easily unless the issue is very dear to my heart.	4	3	3	4
14	I attempt to empower ancillary workers because I find the team spirit is enhanced.	4	3	0	0
15	Personally, I do not really have a vision as to where I plan to be in a few years.	4	3	2	2
16	I enjoy conflict and rarely compromise my needs.	4	3	0	0
17	I am an autonomous person.	4	3	0	0
18	I have been told I am extremely reliable and dependable.	4	3	0	0
19	I have great passion for my nursing career.	4	3	0	0
20	It is important to me to think about and plan for the future.	4	3	0	0

Part 2: Perception of your own ability to lead

Add up your score for Part 2. Here's what the scores indicate:

70 to 80	=	Extremely high perceived leadership ability.
60 to 69	=	High perceived leadership ability.
50 to 59	=	Moderate perceived leadership ability.
40 to 49	=	Low perceived leadership ability.
39 or less	=	Extremely low perceived leadership ability.

LEADERSHIP SKILLS: RATE YOURSELF

Introduction. The best leaders have strengths in at least a half-dozen key emotional-intelligence competencies out of 20 or so. To see how you rate on some of these abilities, assess how the statements below apply to you. Although getting a precise profile of your strengths and weaknesses requires a more rigorous assessment, this quiz can give you a rough rating. More important, we hope it will get you thinking about how well you use leadership skills—and how you might get better at it.

STATEMENT	SEL	OCC	OFT	FREQ
1. I am aware of what I am feeling.				
2. I know my own strengths and weaknesses.				
3. I deal calmly with stress.				
4. I believe the future will be better than the past.				
5. I deal with changes easily.				
6. I set measurable goals when I have a project.				
7. Others say I understand and am sensitive to them.				
8. Others say I resolve conflicts.				
9. Others say I build and maintain relationships.				
10. Others say I inspire them.				
11. Others say I am a team player.				
12. Others say I helped to develop their abilities.				
Total the number of checks in each column:				
	x 1	x 2	x 3	x 4
To get your score, add these four numbers:				
Total Score:				

Interpretation

36 or more = Suggests you are using key leadership skills well—but ask a coworker or partner for his or her opinions, to be more certain.

30–35 = Suggests some strengths but also some underused leadership abilities.

29 or less = Suggests unused leadership abilities and room for improvement.

Leaders are unique, and they can show their talents in different ways. To further explore your leadership strengths, you might ask people whose opinions you value: "When you have seen me do really well as a leader, which of these abilities am I using?" If a number of people tell you that you use the same quality when doing well, you have likely identified a leadership strength that should be appreciated and nurtured.

Source: Goleman, D. (2002). Could you be a leader? *Parade Magazine*, June 16, 2002, pp. 4–6.

References

Bass, B. M. (1990). *Bass and Stogdill's handbook of leadership* (3rd ed.). New York: Free Press.

Bennis, W. (1989). *On becoming a leader*. Reading, MA: Addison-Wesley.

Bennis, W. (2004). A leadership discussion with Warren Bennis. Webcast sponsored by the American Society of Association Executives Foundation, April 20, 2004.

Bennis, W., & Nanus, B. (1985). *Leaders: The strategies for taking charge*. New York: Harper & Row.

Block, P. (1993). *Stewardship: Choosing service over self interest*. San Francisco: Berrett-Koehler.

Bolman, L. G., & Deal, T. E. (2001). *Leading with soul: An uncommon journey of spirit* (New and Revised Ed.). San Francisco: Jossey-Bass.

Burns, J. M. (1978). *Leadership*. New York: Harper Torchbooks.

Burns, J. M. (2003). *Transforming leadership: A new pursuit of happiness.* New York: Atlantic Monthly Press.

Chaleff, I. (1995). *The courageous follower: Standing up to and for our leaders*. San Francisco: Berrett-Koehler.

Clampitt, P. G., & Dekoch, R. J. (2001). *Embracing uncertainty: The essence of leadership.* Armonk, NY: M. E. Sharp.

Collins, J. (2001). Good to great. Retrieved August 8, 2002, from *www.fastcompany.com*

Corona, D. F. (1986). Followership: The indispensable corollary to leadership. In E. C. Hein & M. J. Nicholson (Eds.), *Contemporary leadership behavior: Selected readings* (3rd ed.) (pp. 87–91). Boston: Little, Brown.

DePree, M. (1989). *Leadership is an art*. New York: Dell.

DePree, M. (1992). *Leadership jazz*. New York: Doubleday Currency.

DiRienzo, S. M. (1994). A challenge to nursing: Promoting followers as well as leaders. *Holistic Nursing Practice, 9*(1), 26–30.

Gardner, J. W. (1989). The tasks of leadership. In W. E. Rosenbach & R. L. Taylor (Eds.), *Contemporary issues in leadership* (2nd ed.) (pp. 24–33). Boulder, CO: Westview Press.

Gardner, J. W. (1990). *On leadership*. New York: Free Press.

Greenleaf, R. K. (1977). *Servant leadership: A journey into the nature of legitimate power and greatness.* New York: Paulist Press.

Hesselbein, F., Goldsmith, M., & Somerville, I. (Eds.). (1999). *Leading beyond the walls*. San Francisco: Jossey-Bass.

Holle, M. L., & Blatchley, M. E. (1987). *Introduction to leadership and management in nursing* (2nd ed.). Boston: Jones & Bartlett.

Jackman, I. (Ed.). (2005). *The leader's mentor: Inspiration from the world's most effective leaders.* New York: Random House.

Jennings, B. M., Scalzi, C. C., Rodgers, J. D., & Keane, A. (2007). Differentiating nursing leadership and management competencies. *Nursing Outlook, 55*(4), 169–175.

Kelley, R. (1992). *The power of followership: How to create leaders people want to follow and followers who lead themselves.* New York: Doubleday Currency.

Kelley, R. (1993). How followers weave a web of relationships. In W. E. Rosenbach & R. L. Taylor (Eds.), *Contemporary issues in leadership* (3rd ed.) (pp. 122–133). Boulder, CO: Westview Press.

Kouses, J. M., & Posner, B. Z. (1995). *The leadership challenge: How to keep getting extraordinary things done in organizations.* San Francisco: Jossey-Bass.

Lee, C. (1993). Followership: The essence of leadership. In W. E. Rosenbach & R. L. Taylor (Eds.), *Contemporary issues in leadership* (3rd ed.) (pp. 113–121). Boulder, CO: Westview Press.

Manfredi, C. (1995). The art of legendary leadership. *Nursing Leadership Forum, 1*(2), 62–64.

Nanus, B. (1992). *Visionary leadership.* San Francisco: Jossey-Bass.

Phillips, D. T. (1997). *The founding fathers on leadership.* New York: Warner Books.

Pickens, T. (2000). What makes a good leader? *Creative Living, 29*(4), 13–16.

Spears, L. C. (Ed.). (1995). *Reflections on leadership: How Robert K. Greenleaf's theory of servant-leadership influenced today's top management thinkers.* New York: John Wiley & Sons.

Sturman, C. (2002). Dare to dream. *Leader to Leader, 23*(Winter), 35–39.

Thornberry, N. (2006). A view about "vision." In W. E. Rosenbach & R. L. Taylor (Eds.). *Contemporary issues in leadership* (6th ed.) (pp. 31–43). Boulder, CO: Westview Press.

Tichy, N. M. (1997). *The leadership engine: How winning companies build leaders at every level.* New York: HarperBusiness.

Wheatley, M. J. (1999). *Leadership and the new science: Discovering order in a chaotic world* (2nd ed.). San Francisco: Berrett-Koehler.

Williams, M. (1975). *The velveteen rabbit.* New York: Avon Books.

Yeh, R. T. (2005, November/December). 7 essential qualities of leadership. *Association Executive,* 13.

Zaleznik, A. (1981). Managers and leaders: Are they different? *Journal of Nursing Administration, 11*(7), 25–31.

CHAPTER 2

The World and New Leadership
Changing Our Thinking About Leadership

LEARNING OBJECTIVES
- Define the new leadership that nurses must adopt in order to participate successfully in and shape the healthcare system of today and tomorrow.
- Examine how chaos in our profession currently creates new opportunities for nurses to function as leaders in the healthcare delivery system.
- Describe how each of the following theories are congruent with new perspectives of nursing leadership: chaos, quantum, developmental, cognitive, complexity, and perspective transformation.
- Identify how this new leadership is having a positive impact on the nursing profession, as well as individual nurses.
- Outline strategies to assist nurses' development as new leaders.

INTRODUCTION

Evidence-based practice, patient-centered care, quality and safety, accountability, information management, interdisciplinary collaboration, partnerships, acquisitions, and affiliations; they are terms we hear about, read about, and discuss. All organizations, particularly those in healthcare, are experiencing change. To continue to participate successfully in healthcare, nursing will need to continue to evolve in finding ways to use resources wisely, validate the effects of nursing interventions on patient outcomes, continue to develop strong partnerships, and provide high-quality and cost-effective care.

These goals can be accomplished if we focus on health promotion in all types of care settings, encourage multidisciplinary collaboration, integrate outcome assessment into our daily work as nurses, and "retool," so that nurses can practice even more autonomously and accountably.

To achieve such goals all registered nurses (RNs) and advanced practice nurses (APNs) must think in a whole new way. Being confident as well as competent is consistent with the new view of leadership that nurses will need to have as they solidify their roles in the healthcare arena. Indeed, it is time to embrace the "problems" of organizational change and look at each one of these as a challenging opportunity.

To bring change, a new way of healthcare reform must develop. We are now in a new age of healthcare. A plethora of articles and books discuss the use of unlicensed assistive personnel (UAPs), patient-focused organizational redesign (PFOR), managed care, capitation, the move from illness to health promotion, patient safety, and team building, to name some of the issues. Studies of the effects of these changes on care quality or specific ways in which healthcare providers, especially nurses, need to retool and think in new ways in order to remain significant players in this new age of healthcare are being emphasized (Ewing, 2006; Porter-O'Grady & Malloch, 2007). These studies recommend we change our thinking so that nurses are able to engage in more independent decision-making, collaborate more effectively with nurse and non-nurse partners, and provide leadership (Aiken, Clarke, Sloane, Sochalski, & Siber, 2002; Needleman, Buerhaus, Mattke, Stewart, & Zelevinsky, 2002).

> *Do not follow where the path may lead. Go instead where there is no path and leave a trail.* —Anonymous

PREPARING NURSE LEADERS

Sadly, many nurses are not prepared for the role they will need to assume in acute care institutions, home care, or other settings, and they become overwhelmed all too quickly. This chapter is designed to help nurses rethink the notion of leadership and their roles as leaders, so that they can more effectively participate in the new and ever-evolving healthcare field. In a study by Manfredi and Valiga (1990), a sample of baccalaureate programs was reviewed to evaluate whether the curricula focused more on the art of leadership or on the science of management. These authors found that most of the programs were teaching management. They also reported that faculty generally viewed "leadership" and "management" as synonymous. Thus, there is work to be done if we are to prepare true leaders.

Developing Leadership

We are moving from the Scientific Age with its emphasis on short- and long-term planning, predicting patient acuity, using formulas to provide staff coverage, and following bureaucratic procedures and policies to get tasks done to a New Science Age that stresses empowerment of all, creating while doing, evaluating processes and outcomes, and collaborating as a team. Such change requires us to exercise leadership in an entirely new way.

Covey (2004) described three characteristics a leader must possess for a successful experience in growing and learning: vision, courage, and humility. Having a dream or vision is imperative, but one must have courage to continue to define that vision to a group and, at the same time, be humble enough to know when to redefine it to meet the needs of the changing times and prepare for the future. He also developed the term "co-missioning," which suggests that a staff must not only have a vision or mission but also a way of measuring the outcomes of the vision. This, in turn, will assist in improving the future outcomes. Bennis and Nanus (1995) described leadership as encompassing vision, the ability to communicate effectively, the ability to be steadfast, and the ability to demonstrate positive self-regard. Having the ability to consistently propel a vision in a group or organization takes self-confidence and assertiveness. Parse (1997) echoed the thoughts of Bennis and Nanus when she described leaders as people who are committed to a vision, willing to risk being challenged by others, and demonstrate a reverence for others.

For example, to change our nursing task orientation to a patient outcome focus, nurses can use leadership skills. If our vision was one of nurses working collaboratively with other healthcare members to provide care that best facilitates positive patient outcomes, the monitoring of clients for beneficial or untoward sequelae of nursing, medical, and pharmacological interventions would be done in collaboration with physicians and pharmacists, rather than in isolation of them. Practices that challenge the traditional "sacred cows" of the medical model of practice have to be adopted so that the vision of nursing care taking center stage and nursing being recognized as a primary means to obtaining positive patient outcomes is achieved.

Nursing leaders have been developing nursing diagnoses and a taxonomy of nursing interventions since the 1980s, yet we are still carrying out medical orders. We need to define what nursing is and wants to be, then work as a unified body to achieve those goals. The current chaotic state of healthcare provides a window of opportunity for realization of this vision. (See Chapter 7 for strategies leaders can use to take advantage of these opportunities and to read more in depth about chaos theory.) We need to work to ensure a focus on excellence as well as on the "bottom line." Nursing leaders must clearly identify responsibilities of RNs, APNs, and nonlicensed assistive personnel, and they must guide us in creating and strengthening new roles for nurses. With leaders who employ a new way of thinking about leadership, all of us can be successful in advancing our profession.

CHAOS THEORY

Vicenzi, White, and Begun (1997) suggested nurses take another look at their situations and view them as "complex, dynamic, and unpredictable" (p. 26) rather than as hopeless. These authors acknowledge that nurses are in chaos, as is the entire healthcare system, but chaos theory implies that hidden within this seemingly total disorganization are patterns of order.

"Chaos" is a scientific term meaning "the apparently irregular, unpredictable behavior of deterministic, nonlinear systems" (Vicenzi et al., 1997, p. 26). Wheatley (2006) said computers have awakened us to the true definition of chaos because of their ability to store mega data. Millions of pieces of data can be displayed at any one time on any screen. The system allows the millions of bytes of data to be displayed in what appears to be a chaotic jumble, but as one tracks the computer screen, rapidly moving lines seem to appear and connect the data. Thus, what appeared to be chaos actually takes an orderly shape.

Think about the last time you had an emergency patient situation—didn't everyone pitch in? There were no formalities, and if the patient's situation deteriorated, the team probably became more collegial and informal as everyone tried harder. This is easily correlated to what happens in a bureaucratic organization when uncertainty increases. People tend to use more personal and group approaches (Kouzes & Posner, 1995) as they come together for the *common good*, and this often occurs unconsciously. Leaders can be instrumental at times like this by using the chaos and the changes it ultimately produces as a positive opportunity. In other words, "growth appears from disequilibrium, not balance" (Wheatley, 2006, p. 21).

Challenging problems provide people with opportunities for great success. Sweating a bit or being a little anxious about something usually leaves us exhilarated after the problem has been resolved. The healthcare chaos that currently surrounds us is one such problem. This can result in an even stronger role for nurses and the identification of more creative ways to provide high-quality and cost-effective care. An example may help illustrate this point.

Many in nursing bemoan the loss of the 80% professional staff/20% nonprofessional staff mix we enjoyed in the past and the reality of the current 60% professional staff/40% nonprofessional staff mix in most hospitals today. However, studies such as Needleman, Buerhaus, Stewart, Zelevinsky, and Matki (2006) and Aiken, et al (2002) document that care is better with RN staff, but until it is shown that costs can be maintained with more RN staff, it is unlikely that the proportion of professional staff will increase. It would be contrary to the new science of leadership philosophy, however, to propose a quantitative study measuring cost-effectiveness. Instead, the new science perspective would encourage the emergence of creative leaders who are willing to stray from set formulas and achieve the "right" mix of staff for their individual units by experimenting until that ideal mix is found. For example, a proposal of gradually decreasing professional staff and increasing unlicensed personnel would be more tolerable than just eliminating RN positions. In addition, having an available RN "pool" would allow nurses to be called in when the acuteness of the patient's condition justified professional care. The old bureaucratic way of thinking about having a consistent number of staff members for every unit with a certain number of full-time equivalents (FTEs) of professional and nonprofessional staff, just does not work in a world characterized by chaos.

The new science philosophy recommends less prediction, prejudgment, and compartmentalization. Wheatley (2006, 2005) suggested that we stop dwelling on tasks and instead focus on facilitating the processes needed to obtain desired goals. For example, nurse managers need to try new staffing patterns that acknowledge that a 60% professional and 40% nonprofessional staff mix (or an 80/20, 30/70, or any other mix) is not ideal for every unit, but any number of patterns could work if staff work with each other in new ways. Leaders need to concentrate first on the people who are working to achieve the goals and establishing positive relationships between and among them. Any number of tasks can then be accomplished. If people have positive working relationships with one another, they are more likely to respect one another and to achieve great things. As Wheatley said, "What gives power its charge, positive or negative, is the nature of the relationship" (2006, p. 40).

Some organizations are calling on nurses to navigate their institutions through this chaotic time, and nursing leaders are using a number of creative strategies to influence change, survive, and even grow. Skills such as creativity, patient centeredness, coordination, multiple priority management, problem solving, critical thinking, and system navigation are identified as being necessary for nurses to use throughout their careers. Quantum theory and the new science, developmental theory, cognitive theory, complexity theory, and perspective transformation support a new holistic view of leadership and find growth in chaos. We must come to the realization that chaos is not all bad (Ward, 2001).

QUANTUM THEORY AND THE NEW SCIENCE

Wheatley (2006) was among the first to relate the changes we have witnessed in science to the need for a new view of leadership. She noted that "if we are to continue to draw from science to create and manage organizations, to design research, and to formulate hypotheses about organizational design, planning, economics, human nature, and change processes, then we need to at least ground our work in the science of our times" (p. 8). By "the science of our times," Wheatley is referring to new research in the disciplines of physics, biology, and chemistry, as well as to the theories of chaos and evolution, which span several disciplines. This new science focuses on relationships and a nonlinear approach, in which the real and the potentially real are visualized simultaneously. It is a method of thinking that replaces our standard, orderly, goal-oriented perspective with a free-flowing, open-space, always-moving, anything-can-happen philosophy. Ward (2001) agrees, asserting that "we have been surrounded by order that, until now, physics was unable to explain" (p. 1).

Wheatley (2006) recommended that we approach leadership through the lens provided by the new science and naturally occurring events. For example, after a storm, meteorologists can review storm patterns on a computer and visualize a pattern in what initially appeared to be chaos. We can also reflect on the fact that a stream, which initially seems to be little more than a random collection of water, sand, rocks, and silt, actually is not random at all but is a carefully designed system in which all parts work together to allow flexibility and the capacity for change as the natural elements of storms, animals, and humans affect its path.

The new science says that living systems organize themselves by seeking order, but this order is not linear or predictive. Organizations, said Wheatley (2006), operate in the same way. They seek order, but not in a linear, hierarchical way. Thus, leadership in an organization may best be provided by a social system comprising many leaders, not only one. Those who relate through coercion or with a disregard for others create negative energy, whereas those who are open to others and see others in their fullness create positive energy. Perhaps by focusing on one nonprofessional staff member at a time and allowing a "connectedness" to occur between that individual and the other staff, a we-versus-they situation can be avoided. If each staff member can be empowered to visualize his or her own potential as well as that of each other, a more positive outlook regarding workload and quality of patient care is likely to prevail.

Quantum theory suggests that an interface among all members of a group is critical. Each person needs to be acknowledged for his or her talents and potential, and each needs to be helped to grow. Perhaps we need to visualize the workforce as germinating seeds in space rather than on earth, where gravity pulls the roots toward it and the stem grows away from gravity. In space, seeds grow every which way because there is no gravity to direct them in only a ground-up direction. Likewise, people are not fixed entities gravitating toward one spot and able to be predicted by a set of rules and expectations.

People need to be given the opportunity to grow in all kinds of ways—ways that are unknown to anyone until they happen. It is the task of the leader to encourage and facilitate such growth. Perhaps, visualizing an organization as composed of Gumby-like figures that stretch and overlap with each other in more of a three-dimensional, rather than linear, structure would allow for greater diversity and uniqueness and open more avenues for communication and effective outcomes. Work productivity cannot be predicted based on a given number of FTEs, certain types of patient hours, and acuity levels. Such task-oriented thinking is not what patient care is all about. Instead, our mindsets need to be more multidimensional and open to new possibilities and things that no one has thought of yet. Leaders are the key to success because they facilitate relationships, encourage growth, enjoy uncertainty, and are willing to take risks. Leaders also know how to deal with "toxic" people or those with whom it is difficult to communicate, develop outstanding leaders, and transform organizations (Porter-O'Grady & Malloch, 2007).

The new way of thinking about leadership in a global and almost limitless fashion, and realizing that each individual has a contribution to make, is necessary if nursing is to succeed in delivering the highest-quality care. Valuing hard work and respecting one another are values that need to be revived and that must be pervasive. In other words, the whole culture of our practice settings needs reawakening. A job should be viewed as a piece of an ever-changing plan that affects the overall functioning of the organization. Each person must be respected as crucial to the greater goal. Biases, prejudices, insecurities, and preconceived judgments need to be worked out or left behind. When such an atmosphere exists, communication, mentoring, and collaboration are more likely to occur, and self-empowerment and group empowerment dominate. The change from a task-focused setting to more of a process-focused one allows followers and leaders to propel organizations and the individuals within them forward.

The world is moving out of the Industrial or Newtonian Age in which things were described in a linear way and where we became accustomed to separating every system into parts, rather than dealing with the whole. As the world moves toward this greater concern for wholeness, complexity, and interaction, leaders are needed. An example of a healthcare organization being more process-focused and implementing an holistic approach to leadership is provided in the accompanying case study.

We must use our imaginations and embrace the idea that there is more to our work than assessing, planning, implementing, and evaluating. Nurses can no longer have tunnel vision and be task-oriented. Instead, we need a more in-depth analysis

New Science of Leadership Case Study

The senior leadership at an acute care institution were working on more integration of the six issues delineated by the Institute of Medicine's *Crossing the Quality Chasm – A New Health System for the 21st Century* (2001), which include patient safety, patient-centeredness, efficiency, effectiveness, timeliness, and equity. One of the nurse leader executives suggested the development of a Patient/Family Advisory Board, which would allow volunteers who served on this Board to be integrated into the infrastructure of the hospital. This would entail representatives from this Patient/Family Advisory Board sitting in on the hospital's executive leadership sessions, the Hospital Governing Board meetings, and other similar group discussions with an aim toward setting a new standard of care in order to obtain a meaningful voice for patients and families. The nurse leader, the vice president of patient outcomes, marketed the idea, sought volunteers from the community, established the Board, assisted in developing bylaws for the board, integrated the board members into the hospital's organization, and now meets monthly with the board and other groups to receive feedback. Members of the Patient/Family Advisory Board include previous hospital patients and family members of patients who had been hospitalized or died. The outcomes are assisting in promoting a patient safety culture to advance optimum care by establishing priorities, developing specific action plans, and allocating appropriate resources. The Joint Commission and the Institute for Healthcare Improvement recognize that effective leadership is essential toward creating a safe and patient-centered care delivery system (Aspden, Corrigan, Wolcott, & Erickson, 2004; Institute for Healthcare Improvement, 2007). This is a most innovative way to ensure a meaningful voice is provided to healthcare consumers.

of the data collected before we can decide on what to include in the plan of care. Our whole philosophy of caring for patients must be broadened, and for most of us, our way of simply moving from one task to another will have to change. Most RNs, the average of whom is 42.3 years old and has worked most of her or his 20-plus-year career in a very rigid organizational structure carrying out another profession's orders, will have to reorient themselves to nursing and to leading with a new science of leadership perspective. The quantum mechanics framework of attending to naturally occurring events appreciates individuals for their knowledge and recognizes that they need tools and support, not direction and control (Malloch & Porter-O'Grady, 2005).

SUPPORTING PERSPECTIVES AND PERSPECTIVE TRANSFORMATION THEORY

The idea that people and organizations grow and evolve in response to challenges, disequilibrium, and change is not new, nor is it restricted to quantum mechanics or new science thinking. In fact, it is an idea that has been addressed by psychologists, educators, and nurse theorists. Examples of these follow.

Cognitive and intellectual development occur as one is increasingly able to use complex cognitive skills to analyze issues, manage changing circumstances, integrate multiple points of view, and make sound decisions independently (Perry, 1970). Individuals progress through stages of cognitive development, from seeing knowledge as finite and themselves as absorbers or memorizers of it, to viewing knowledge as relative and themselves as critical thinkers and lifelong learners. Such changes in worldview, similar to any type of growth, occur as a result of disequilibrium. When one's usual way of thinking is found to be lacking, one experiences disequilibrium and is challenged to think in new ways, ask new questions, and develop new strategies. The chaos and disequilibrium with which nurses in practice are challenged, therefore, can be viewed as a stimulus for growth and development. Nurses need to rethink their role in healthcare, the kind of leadership needed in this arena, and their responsibility to provide such leadership.

Erik Erikson, a developmental theorist, stated that physical, emotional, and social factors have an effect on an individual's development (Erikson, 1963). He asserted that development is a mixture of maturation (the potential growth a person has inherited) and learning (knowledge to be gained). Most nurses are working in a rigidly structured healthcare system and, without leadership, may not move out of adolescence or young adulthood stages, where one of the tasks is to master involvement with others. Mastery of these developmental tasks results in intimacy and solidarity, whereas failure results in isolation. Since the new leadership is based on relationships, it is paramount that nurses accomplish the task of young adulthood, so that they can be highly effective healthcare team members. The accomplishment of the generativity task (Erickson, 1963) for those more advanced in life leads to productive and creative work. For nurses to experience this generativity, they need to have acquired leadership skills.

Just as our lives can be viewed developmentally, so too can our organizational systems. Only organizational structures that continue to be flexible and change will be able to support the development of people in the organization. Sometimes, it is only when a person is pushed, as happens in a chaotic job setting or in severe conflict with one's peers to accomplish tasks, does he or she actually develop and grow. Hence, developmental theory also suggests that disequilibrium is not a negative thing, but rather a positive experience that enhances growth.

Complexity theory describes the way life is ordered and stresses that life is based on the principles of emergence more so than predetermined by other variables. McDaniel and Driebe (2005) explore how unpredictability and surprise affect our world both individually and through our various group classifications. The ideas of how complexity science influences everything we do, including leading, are explained by West (2006), who gives multiple examples of how emergence, self-organization, and pattern formation underlie the science of complexity.

Fawcett (1995) explained that "each nurse, as well as the healthcare system itself, requires time to evolve from the use of individual, implicit frames of reference for nursing practice to an explicit model" (p. 532). The process that occurs during this period of growth, when an individual has not clearly defined a frame of reference for nursing practice to a clearly defined conceptual model, is perspective transformation. This growth depends on the experiences one has had in school or in the work setting. Using Fawcett's (1995, pp. 533–534) explanation of perspective transformation, one can visualize how leaders can assist nurses to identify their own ability to lead and hence grow in these chaotic times.

> *Stage 1: Stability* reflects what many nurses are currently experiencing in their workplaces. Nurses easily maintain the status quo because many were never encouraged to think of themselves as leaders.
>
> *Stage 2: Dissonance* moves one toward the revelation that all nurses can be leaders. It generally means the beginning of a reawakening to one's situation. Nurses experiencing dissonance are aware of the very chaotic times they are in and know they need to start doing something. They may share their feelings with peers and start speaking out when serious staffing problems or unsafe situations occur.

Stage 3: Confusion occurs when individuals gain courage from others who validate what they are feeling, speak openly about things not being right, and decide not to "put up with it anymore!"

Stage 4: Dealing with uncertainty is when individuals speak out, but they do so sporadically because they may believe that they do not have the ability or strength to change things.

Stage 5: Saturation occurs when people feel confident they have collected the right information and spoken to the right people about a new way of doing things or delivering care.

Stage 6: Synthesis heralds the organization of information to formulate a plan to change an unacceptable situation . . . a plan put into place because individuals cared enough to make a change.

Stage 7: Resolution indicates that the problems are being solved with the changes that were put into place.

Stage 8: Reconceptualization occurs when those who initiated the change continue to "work out some of the kinks" in the system and empower others to continue to support and pursue new ways of doing things.

Stage 9: Return to stability indicates that the change has now become a part of the milieu and is no longer being evaluated and scrutinized extensively.

This framework provides an additional basis for arguing why we need to rethink the need for leadership. It depicts a change from nurses practicing in a private way to an entire nursing staff using a shared model of practice. This is a good example of how something positive can come from living or working in chaos. Perspective transformation is a helpful process to use in assisting nurses to practice more autonomously. It could also facilitate nursing receiving a greater portion of the healthcare dollar because it should assist in measuring tangible patient outcomes, which are a direct result of nursing care.

CONCLUSION

We need to change our thinking about what leadership is if we are to survive and thrive during the tumultuous changes in healthcare. Chaos theory will assist us in understanding how the disorder and confusion we are feeling in our work settings today are equivalent to what happens in nature. The fact that the natural world we live in can automatically order itself after such turmoil is incredible. We have to realize that adapting the new science of leadership, with its focus on empowering followers and alleviating the bureaucratic organizational structure, will assist us in developing new ideas and new ways of working.

The transformation to managed care that nurses have confronted is certainly disorienting and chaotic, but it is necessary to change the hierarchical medical model on which the U.S. healthcare system has been based. This major paradigm shift has the potential to improve the quality of healthcare and not merely reduce costs. That will happen, however, only if we have capable leaders willing to take the risks needed to produce such positive outcomes. Quantum theory, cognitive theory, developmental theory, complexity theory, and perspective transformation frameworks provide evidence that chaos and disequilibrium can be positive instigators for growth and improvement. This new way of thinking about leading will help nurses provide a more collaborative and holistic approach to practice and help us achieve our visions for the profession.

CRITICAL THINKING EXERCISES

Explain how the new way of thinking about leadership described in this chapter can affect the way we conceptualize the role of the nurse today. How could you assist others in adapting this perspective?

_____

_____

Think about the environment in which you practice. Would you describe it as chaotic? Why or why not? What contributes to the chaos or relative "calm"? What have been the negative ways that you and others have dealt with chaos in your environment? What positive strategies have been used? What patterns do you see in the midst of all this chaos?

_____

_____

Listen to a jazz musical selection with an extended improvisational piece. Despite the seemingly chaotic notes and chords, do you hear or feel any patterns or synchrony? How did you identify such patterns? (Note: This same exercise can be done by viewing a later Picasso painting, or even watching a soccer game.)

_____

_____

Who do you think of as leaders where you practice? What characteristics of the new science of leadership do these people portray?

_____

_____

Develop a list of behaviors that you use when you approach various situations regarding certainty or uncertainty. Describe how your work environment (the people and the structure) influences your certainty.

_____

_____

_____

References

Aiken, L., Clarke, S., Sloane, D., Sochalski, J., & Siber, J. (2002). Hospital staffing and patient mortality, nurse burnout, and job dissatisfaction. *Journal of the American Medical Association, 288,* 1987–1993.

Aspden, P., Corrigan, J., Wolcott, J., & Erickson, S. (Eds.). (2004). *Patient safety: Achieving a new standard for care.* Washington, DC: National Academy of Sciences.

Bennis, W., & Nanus, B. (1995). *Leadership: The strategies for taking charge.* New York: Harper & Row.

Clampitt, H., & DeKoch, R. (2001). *Embracing uncertainty: The essence of leadership.* Armonk, NY: M. E. Sharpe.

Covey, S. (2004). *The 8th habit: From effectiveness to greatness.* New York: Free Press.

Erikson, E. (1963). *Childhood and society* (2nd ed.). New York: W. W. Norton.

Ewing, B. (2006). A quantum leap for leadership. *Nursing Spectrum, 16*(17), 29.

Fawcett, J. (1995). *Analysis and evaluation of conceptual models of nursing* (3rd ed.). Philadelphia: F.A. Davis.

Institute of Healthcare Improvement. (2007). *100K lives campaign.* Accessed July 17, 2007, from *www.ihi.org/IHI/Programs/Campaign*

Institute of Medicine. (2001). *Crossing the quality chasm: New health system for the 21st century.* Washington, DC: The National Academies Press.

Kouzes, J., & Posner, B. (1995). *The leadership challenge: How to keep getting extraordinary things done in organizations* (2nd ed.). San Francisco: Jossey-Bass.

Malloch, K., & Porter-O'Grady, T. (2005). *The quantum leader: Applications for the new world of work.* Sudbury, MA: Jones & Bartlett.

Manfredi, C., & Valiga, T. (1990). How are we preparing nurse leaders? A study of baccalau- reate curriculum. *Journal of Nursing Education, 29*(1), 4–9.

McDaniel, R., & Driebe, D. (Eds.). (2005). *Uncertainty and surprise in complex systems.* New York: Springer.

Needleman, J., Buerhaus, P., Mattke, S., Stewart, M., & Zelevinsky, K. (2002). Nurse-staffing levels and the quality of care in hospitals. *New England Journal of Medicine, 346*(22), 1715–1722.

Needleman, J., Buerhaus, P., Stewart, M., Zelevinsky, K., & Matke, S. (2006). Is there a busi- ness case for quality? *Health Affairs, 25*(1), 204–211.

Parse, R. (1997). Leadership: The essentials. (Editorial). *Nursing Science Quarterly, 10*(3), 109.

Perry, W. (1970). *Forms of intellectual and ethical development in the college years: A scheme.* New York: Holt, Rinehart, & Winston.

Porter-O'Grady, T., & Malloch, K. (2007). *Quantum leadership: A resource or health care inno- vation* (2nd ed.). Sudbury, MA: Jones & Bartlett.

Vicenzi, A., White, K., & Begun, J. (1997). Chaos in nursing: Make it work for you. *American Journal of Nursing, 97*(10), 26–32.

Ward, M. (2001). *Beyond chaos: The underlying theory behind life, the universe, and everything*. New York: Thomas Dunce Books.

West, B. (2006). *Where medicine went wrong: Rediscovering the path to complexity*. Hackensack, NJ: World Scientific Publishing Co. Inc.

Wheatley, M. (2005). *Finding our way: Leadership for an uncertain time*. San Francisco: Berrett-Koehler Publishers, Inc.

Wheatley, M. (2006). *Leadership and the new science: Discovering order in a chaotic world* (3rd ed.). San Francisco: Berrett-Koehler Publishers, Inc.

CHAPTER 3

Followership and Empowerment

LEARNING OBJECTIVES
- Examine the similarities between leaders and followers.
- Articulate the interdependence between leaders and followers.
- Describe sources of power.
- Examine how power can be used to empower oneself and others.
- Formulate strategies to develop oneself as an effective follower.

INTRODUCTION

In today's socio-technical organizations, the culture is collective ("team"), the expectation is involvement and investment, and the style of implementation is facilitative and integrative —(Porter-O'Grady, 1993, p.53).

In today's flatter, leaner environment, organizations and leaders cannot succeed without committed, contributing followers —(Kelley, 1992, p. 200).

With the kind of organizational environments described here, it is clear that leaders will need to work collaboratively with followers if any group or organization is to succeed. Indeed, "any organization is a triad consisting of leaders and followers joined in a common purpose . . . Followers and leaders orbit around the purpose; followers do not orbit around the leader" (Chaleff, 1995, p. 11) (Fig. 3–1). Despite this need for collaboration, however, we know very little about followers and followership even though we are coming to know more and more about leaders and leadership.

Leadership and followership are two separate concepts, two separate roles that are complementary or reciprocal, not competitive (Barwick, 2007). They are synergistic, "a dialectic . . . depend[ing] on each other for existence and meaning" (Kelley, 1992, p. 45). In other words, just as "up" has little meaning were it not for "down," the word "leader" has little meaning without the word "follower," and vice versa. In fact, "there can be no leaders without followers" (Goffee & Jones, 2006, p. 127), and there can be no followers without leaders.

No one person can know the best strategy, have the clearest vision, or identify the most effective approaches to solve problems. Indeed, "none of us is as smart as all of us" (Bennis, 2006, p. 136). Thus, "all participants [need to be] recognized as full partners in the organizational venture . . . [and they need to be] co-leaders in the enterprise" (Sullivan, 1998, p. 469).

As a duality relationship, leaders must understand that people seek, admire, respect and follow those who let them know they are important and significant, who create a sense of community, and who create environments that produce a "buzzing feeling" (Goffee & Jones, 2006, p. 128), characterized by excitement, challenge, and a sense of engagement, where people feel they are part of something larger or more important than themselves. Organizations of today and the future need "a new, more democratic vision [that] . . . creates dynamic partnerships, combining the best of what we are collectively while empowering us as individuals" (Dreher, 1996, p. xiii), particularly since the "freedom to uncover new ideas and create an environment that encourages followers to share their best thinking with their leaders is essential to innovation and change" (Potter & Rosenbach, 2006, p. 143).

The leadership expert, Warren Bennis (2004, p. 1), asserts, "The longer I study effective leaders, the more I am convinced of the underappreciated importance of effective followers." He also claims that "in our society leadership is too often seen as an inherently individual phenomenon" (Bennis, 2006, p. 130) but acknowledges that "no change can occur without willing and committed followers" (p. 133). Thus, both leaders and followers are increasingly important (Fig. 3–2).

Old Conceptualization of Leader-Follower Interactions

Contemporary Conceptualizations of Leader-Follower Interactions

FIGURE 3–1 • Old and contemporary conceptualizations of leader-follower interactions.

FIGURE 3–2 • Leaders need followers.

> *The secret of leadership is . . . the ability to inspire others with faith in their own high potential.*
>
> —J. Donald Walters

As many have noted, *leaders can be leaders only if they have followers.* Indeed, "to be a leader means generating followership" (Staub, 1996, p. 74) and "followership is the basis for all leadership" (Staub, 1996, p. 76). One author (Lundy, 1993, p. 21) flatly stated that "the ultimate criterion [in defining] a leader . . . is anyone who has followers." Despite these assertions, however, the concept of followership is rarely addressed to the same extent as the concept of leadership. No conferences are held about followership. Individuals do not seek consultation on how to be an effective follower. There is little, if any, content in educational programs on effective followership, and little has been written on the concept. Why does such a significant role receive so little attention? Does our emphasis on leadership "compensate for something in our culture or our organizations that fills us with an exaggerated need to promote leadership and to silence whatever haunts us about the notion of followership?" (Berg, 1998, p. 28).

> *The final test of a leader is that he leaves behind him in other men the conviction and the will to carry on.*
>
> —Walter Lippman

Few would argue that followership is a neglected topic. In fact, a recent review of textbooks on nursing leadership and management (Anderson, 1999; Rocchiccioli & Tilbury, 1998; Swansburg & Swansburg, 2002; Yoder-Wise, 2003) revealed virtually no mention of the concept. In a seminal book titled *Strategies for the Future of Nursing* (O'Neil & Coffman, 1998), little mention is made of leadership and none of followership.

In one nursing leadership and management book, the word "follower" was used only as an example of a role someone in a group often takes to build and maintain the group. Follower was defined as "a group member who accepts the other group members' ideas and listens to their discussion and decisions" (Swansburg & Swansburg, 1999, p. 402). In this same book, the authors talked about the mutual influence of leaders and those they lead; however, the authors chose to use the word "constituent" instead of "follower." Although they did not provide the reader with a reason for the choice of words, one might assume it has something to do with the negative connotations the word "follower" often carries.

In her review of her own path to leadership as the president of the American Nurses' Association, Joel (1999) said she was an "extraordinary follower . . . [who] learned the rules well and followed them exactly . . . [who was] too intimidated to question authority . . . [and who] lacked confidence" (p. 17). She was, in essence, invisible.

One might conclude from these brief examples that there is something about the word "follower" or the notion of followership that is negative, demeaning, and unattractive. In reality, however, the follower role is a powerful one because "the responsibility for making the leader-follower relationship work remains with the 'follower'" (Berg, 1998, p. 33).

THE CONCEPT OF FOLLOWERSHIP

Being a "good" follower takes special talents, just as being a "good" leader does. Indeed, the qualities of leaders and followers are very similar. Thus, conscious attention must be given to the development of followers and followership must be cultivated, just as leadership development and the cultivation of leadership are important. If we fail to remember that followership is voluntary, fail to convey the importance of followership, and fail to cultivate effective followers, leaders will be left without the support needed to realize visions, make change, and create a preferred future. In essence, when the cry goes out to "follow the leader," few will know who to follow or how to follow, and little will be accomplished. Worse yet, the masses will not be prepared to identify the worthy leader and may follow the person with the loudest voice or the most charisma, as was the case with the Hitler Youth, the Jim Jones Guyana community, and the Waco, Texas, commune.

"Being willing to follow is not about blindly accepting some new leader's authority, nor expecting that they will have all the answers at the outset. It's also not about abdicating all responsibility for progress and getting things done or waiting passively for the answers to be provided on a plate by the leader and deciding that you'll change when some results start to occur. Nor is it about sitting back and hoping to enjoy the ride" (DiCarlo, 2002, p. 2). Effective followers are much more active and involved than this.

Followership is an art—a skill that can be learned, cultivated, and consciously developed and exercised. Followers need to be "self-directing, actively participating, practicing experts [who work] on behalf of the organization and the mutually agreed upon vision and goals" (Sullivan, 1998, p. 469). They need to trust others and be trustworthy themselves. They need to see themselves as a community, think and act as a team, and invest energy in team building by focusing on the common goal and drawing on the strengths and talents of each member of the team. Followers need to know their own strengths and what their unique contributions to the effort can be. They must complement each other's and the leader's specialties, strengths, and areas of expertise. They need to seek information so that they have the "larger picture," which allows them to participate fully and provide significant feedback. Followers should not invest their energy merely in their own or others' individual or personal agendas. They also should not ally themselves with group members whose goals are out of alignment with those of the rest of the team. They need to be counted on to "provide input that focuses on finding solutions, not just on articulating problems" (Sullivan, 1998, p. 478). They are expected to support the leader by asking questions, giving thoughtful feedback, working to achieve group goals, and providing encouragement when the leader takes a risk on behalf of the group (Corona, 1986); leaders, in return, are expected to support followers by seeking their input, using their talents fully, and encouraging them to grow continually. Leaders and followers must "fuse to move together toward a common goal" (Joel, 1999, p. 30).

> *The secret of leadership is . . . never to ask of others what you would not willingly do yourself.*
> —*J. Donald Walters*

Followership also involves knowing when and how to assume the role of leader when necessary. "The organization is essentially a community of many leaders and many followers, frequently changing places depending on the particular activity that is occurring" (Sullivan, 1998, p. 477). "We all have the capacity to become either leaders or followers and both are necessary. There are no leaders without followers, and no matter how high you climb the leadership ladder, there is always the requirement to follow some of the time . . . These roles are not in competition, but rather natural compliments [*sic*] to one another's success" (Joel, 1999, p. 29).

It has been asserted that followers, simply by being in the presence of a leader and feeling how that individual does what she/he does, will take on the necessary abilities to move toward realization of the vision (Goldsmith, 2007). Thus, leaders need to step aside and allow followers to take the lead in the group when their abilities, passions, and perspectives are more appropriate to the situation (Salacuse, 2005).

A follower is an individual who takes another as a role model and who acts in accordance with, imitates, supports and advocates the ideas and opinions of another (Brown, 1980). Without both leaders and followers, "there can be no unity, no successful goal-directed activity, and no true . . . achievement" (Brown, 1980, p. 357). But "taking another as a role model," "imitating," and "acting in accordance with another" do not mean that followers are passive, unthinking individuals who have no ideas of their own. On the contrary, "supporting and advocating the ideas and opinions of another" demand that the follower think critically about those ideas and opinions, have the skills to advocate for those ideas, and take an active role in providing support to the leader as the ideas are fully developed and advanced. The following case study illustrates the powerful role followers play.

Case Study

Helen is a staff RN in a long-term care facility whose resident population averages 80 years of age. She has read research that shows increased family involvement in the care of the elderly helps decrease their confusion and increase their participation in self-care activities. For the past month, Helen has provided leadership among her colleagues to find more ways to increase family involvement, and positive results are being observed. While Helen feels encouraged by those outcomes and takes pride in knowing they are the result of her vision and leadership efforts, the realization that the positive results are limited to a very few residents is disappointing. Knowing that more individuals could benefit from the intervention, Helen encourages other staff to brainstorm about how to increase the involvement of more families. Several CNAs who have worked closely with the residents over time offer perspectives that Helen had not considered and suggest changes in the ideas Helen had proposed initially. Colleagues in dietary, physical therapy, and social services support these new ideas and add to them. Helen appreciates the value of these suggestions from those who had been following her lead and, together, the team designs a "menu" of ways actual or surrogate family members can participate more actively in the care of all residents on the unit.

The secret of leadership is . . . inviting cooperation from others, rather than demanding their obedience.
—J. Donald Walters

TYPES OF FOLLOWERS

Despite the vital role that followers actually play in effecting change and realizing visions, many still see the role as passive, dependent, unthinking, and lacking in status. Such negative perceptions of followers and followership are common, but they suggest that there is only one type of follower. Kelley (1992, 1998), on the other hand, suggests that there are several types of followers (Fig. 3–3), ranging from those who are vital to the success of the group or organization to those who are passive and unthinking:

- *Effective or exemplary followers:* These individuals function independently, think critically about ideas that are proposed or directions that are suggested, and are actively involved. They challenge the ideas of the leader, suggest alternative courses of action, and invest time and energy to arrive at the best possible solution for the group.
- *Alienated followers:* These individuals think critically about what the leader or other members of the group are suggesting, but they remain passive and perhaps even somewhat hostile. They may complain about "the way things are being done," are unhappy, and seem disengaged at times. Alienated followers will rarely invest time or energy to suggest alternative solutions or other approaches.
- *Yes people:* These are the conformists who are actively involved in the work of the group and enthusiastically support the leader. They are eager to take orders, defer to the leader, yield to the leader's views and opinions, and please the leader. They enjoy a great deal of structure, order, and predictability. "Yes" people are uncomfortable with having

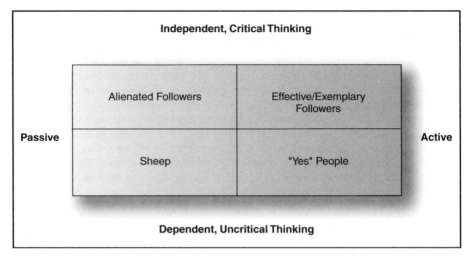

Independent, Critical Thinking

Alienated Followers	Effective/Exemplary Followers
Sheep	"Yes" People

Passive · Active

Dependent, Uncritical Thinking

FIGURE 3–3 • Types of followers. (Adapted from Kelley, R.E. [1998]. In praise of followers. In W. E. Rosenbach & R. L. Taylor [Eds.], *Contemporary issues in leadership* [4th ed.] [p. 98]. Boulder, CO: Westview Press; and Kelley, R. [1992]. *The power of followership: How to create leaders people want to follow and followers who lead themselves* [p. 97]. New York: Doubleday Currency.)

to make and live with decisions, and they find freedom almost terrifying. They do not initiate ideas, think for themselves, raise questions, critique the ideas of others, or challenge the group.

• **Sheep:** These are the passive individuals who are dependent and uncritical, going along with whatever the leader tells them to do. They are easily led and manipulated, lack initiative, require a great deal of direction, and never go beyond their given assignment. "Sheep" are not particularly committed to the goals of the group and do not invest themselves to any great extent to see that the group continues to move forward.

Types of followers, or followership styles, have also been described by Pittman, Rosenbach, and Potter (1998). Rather than using Kelley's (1992, 1998) "passive/active" and "independent/dependent" parameters, these authors use the dimensions of "performance initiative" and "relationship initiative" to define four followership styles (Fig. 3–4).

Performance initiatives relate to the follower's performance—how his or her assigned job gets done, how good the person is at what he or she does, the standards the person sets for himself or herself, how well the person works with others, and how valuable the person is to the organization. *Relationship initiatives* concern the follower's relationship to the leader—how much the person understands the leader's perspective, the person's willingness to give negative feedback or disagree with the leader, and how the person demonstrates his or her reliability and trustworthiness. Each of the four followership styles reflects extensive or limited activity in these dimensions:

• **Partner:** This follower is committed to high performance and building a positive, reciprocal relationship with the leader. The partner may be

Performance Initiative

	Politician	Partner	**High**
Relationship Initiatives	Subordinate	Contributor	**Low**
	Low	**High**	

FIGURE 3–4 • Followership styles. (Source: Pittman, T. S., Rosenbach, W. E., & Potter, E. H., III. [1998]. Followers as partners: Taking the initiative for action. In W. E. Rosenbach & R. L. Taylor [Eds.], *Contemporary issues in leadership* [4th ed.] [p. 113]. Boulder, CO: Westview Press.)

thought of as a "leader-in-waiting" (Pittman, Rosenbach & Potter, 1998, p. 118).

- **Contributor:** This person does the job very well, is effective with coworkers, embraces change, and successfully balances work and other aspects of life. The contributor does not, however, try to understand the leader's perspective or promote the leader's vision, nor does he or she negotiate differences maturely, communicate courageously, share her/his expertise and knowledge, or take initiative (Chaleff, 1995; Pittman, Rosenbach, & Potter, 1998; Potter & Rosenbach, 2006).
- **Politician:** This individual is highly sensitive to and skilled with interpersonal relationships. The person is willing to give honest feedback and supports the leader; however, he or she may neglect the job and have poor performance levels.
- **Subordinate:** This type of follower may be competent at assigned tasks and do what he or she is told, but there is no commitment to excellence in his or her performance. In addition, the subordinate is not particularly sensitive to relationships, does not make an effort to support the leader, is disaffected, and is not interested in giving anything extra (Potter & Rosenbach, 2006).

One other way to think about types of followers was offered by DiCarlo (2002), who outlined the "5-P Follower Model." This author identified five types of followers: *Participants*, who are actively involved and contribute to moving the group forward; *Pessimists*, who think any change is bad and share that perspective with everyone; *Passengers*, those individuals who are in the group in body, but not necessarily in mind or heart; *Pigs,* those who are involved only for the benefits they can reap person-ally; and *Prisoners,* who participate but not through choice.

Regardless of the model used to think about types of followers, each type often can often be identified by the behaviors exhibited (Potter & Rosenbach, 2006). Consider the follower's active efforts to do a good job, including actual performance, effective-ness in working with others, serving as a resource for others, and the extent to which change is embraced. One also can examine the follower's working relationship with the leader, including the extent to which one identifies with the leader, active attempts to strengthen the relationship, efforts to build and sustain trust, the ability to negotiate differences, and the willingness to engage in "courageous conversations" (Potter & Rosenbach, 2006, p. 152) where the follower is honest, may disagree with the leader, and takes risks.

What nursing needs as we participate in and, indeed, work to shape today's health-care arena are effective or exemplary followers, partners, or participants. We need people who can support even small changes in practice or behavior that then become the new norm, a process referred to as the "normalization of deviation" (Kohn, Corrigan, & Donaldson, 2000, p. 55). Blindly following some leader without question or taking a passive role in one's work setting, community, or professional organization will do little to advance the profession, promote individual growth, and achieve quality patient care. Instead, nursing needs followers who have characteristics that are similar to those of leaders: a willingness to serve, assertiveness, determination, a will-ingness to challenge ideas, courage, an ability to act as a change agent, and an open-ness to new ideas and perspectives. Indeed, followers and leaders must complement each other (Corona, 1986), as noted in Table 3–1.

CHARACTERISTICS OF EFFECTIVE OR EXEMPLARY FOLLOWERS

Although the term "follower" often "conjures up images of docility, conformity, weakness, and failure to excel" (Chaleff, 1995, p. 3), effective or exemplary followers

TABLE 3-1 Traits of Leaders and Followers

LEADERS	FOLLOWERS
Study and create new ideas.	Test new ideas.
Make decisions.	Challenge decisions as needed.
Assign appropriate responsibilities.	Know when to accept responsibility and do so.
Create environments of trust, resulting in freedom.	Use freedom responsibly.
Take risks.	Risk following.
Are reliable.	Are trustworthy and respectful.
Are loyal to the followers.	Are loyal to the leader.
Are self-confident.	Know themselves.
Assume the leadership position.	Follow when appropriate.

possess many of the same characteristics as those individuals who exercise leadership. Each of us may do well to reflect on the extent to which we are characterized by the following:

- Strength and independence
- Critical thinking
- Ability and willingness to think for ourselves
- Ability to give honest feedback and constructive criticism, particularly in a timely fashion
- Willingness to be our own person
- Innovativeness and creativity
- Active engagement in all we do
- Cooperativeness and collaborativeness
- Being a self-starter
- "Going above and beyond the call of duty"— beyond our job assignments
- Willingness to assume ownership
- Taking initiative
- Positive sense of self-worth
- "Can do" aura (Kelley, 1992, p. 143)
- Attentiveness to what is happening around us
- "Holding up our end of the bargain"
- Being energized by our work and organization(s)

Through his work with workshop participants, Berg (1998) identified additional characteristics of exemplary followers. He described these individuals as "interesting characters" (p. 40) who were bold and colorful—not passive or bland—loyal, and supportive. They possessed their own distinctive voices that leaders typically heeded well. Exemplary followers openly expressed their own ideas, concerns, perspectives, and even conflicting views, and effective leaders paid attention to these voices. A nurse who proposes to the nurse manager and colleagues how family members can be more involved in planning and, indeed, coordinating or directing the care of patients with serious illnesses—when that is not the norm on the unit—is being bold, not passive, and expressing conflicting views. The colleagues who take this suggestion seriously and consider changing the practice standards on the unit are enriched by this nurse's proposal, and the ultimate goal toward which they are all working—quality patient and family care—is more likely to be realized.

Berg (1998) also found that an emotional connection exists between leaders and exemplary followers, a relation he suggested may be needed so that each can reassure the other "during those times when each must show his or her limits and weaknesses to the other" (p. 41). For example, the nurse manager who has been unsuccessful in securing additional staff positions so that nurses can attend valuable in-service programs and participate in grand rounds needs to be able to express that frustration. Likewise, staff need to be able to acknowledge when they do not have the knowledge or skill to care for a particular patient. Showing one's limitations and weaknesses requires a mutual trust, a bond, and an emotional connection between the leader and the followers.

> *Power wins, not by being used, but by being there.*
> —*Anonymous*

Effective followers, then, are far from being invisible and clones of leaders. Instead, they actually stimulate and inspire leaders, challenge their creativity, collaborate with them, complement them, give them feedback, and support them. Leaders may inspire vision, but it is the followers who supply much of the energy to achieve that vision. Indeed, followership is "the important phenomenon to study if we are to understand why organizations succeed or fail" (Kelley, 1992, p. 5).

Followers assume such an active role, however, only when they get what they expect from leaders, and what they expect is credibility (Kouzes & Posner, 1993). Followers want leaders who are *honest*—individuals who are consistent, ethical, and principled. They want leaders who are *competent*—who know their field of endeavor and know the work that needs to be done. They want leaders who are *inspiring*—individuals who are enthusiastic, contagious, visionary, and effective in communicating a dream. And, they want leaders who are *forward looking*—oriented toward the "big picture" and able to help followers see their important place in that picture. We might think of these factors in terms of a formula for successful leadership and effective leader-follower relations:

Honesty + Competence + Inspiration + Vision = Credibility

Leaders and followers are interdependent. Theirs is a reciprocal relationship, and they reinforce each other. Indeed, the qualities of leaders and followers are so closely aligned that one could assume that the same people who are seen by their peers as desirable leaders would also be seen as desirable followers. Individuals often move back and forth between leader and follower roles, depending on the situation. They draw on the same skills to be effective in either role. Both have power, but where does that power come from, and how do leaders and followers use it to empower themselves and others?

SOURCES OF POWER

Leadership has sometimes been referred to as a power relationship, and Bass (1990) asserted that one cannot lead without power. Thus, part of the leadership process is the ability to use power, not control, to influence the direction of the group and realization of the vision.

> *Power and influence can be wielded with grace and authority, even when results must be delivered without fail.* —*Nancy Austin*

Oftentimes we think of power negatively, conjuring up images of exploitation and manipulation. Those in authority may abuse the power of their positions when allowing personal feelings for or against a staff member, for example, to influence staffing assignments, performance evaluations, or the awarding of "perks" or benefits (time off to attend a conference, serving as a preceptor). Power, however, does not derive only from one's position of authority.

In 1960, French and Raven published a seminal work in which they identified five sources of power:

> **Legitimate power** comes from one's title or position, or role in a family or culture.
>
> **Coercive power** comes from the ability to penalize others. For example, in his discourses on freedom in the first century A.D., Epictetus said, "No one is afraid of Caesar himself, but he is afraid of death, loss of property, prison, [and] disengagement."
>
> **Reward power** comes from the ability to help and get things (e.g., money, praise) for others.
>
> **Expert power** comes from one's knowledge or competence.
>
> **Referent power** comes from followers' respect for and their desire to be liked and admired by the leader. As Reed (2004) notes, "There is inherently more power and leverage in serving your [followers] versus them attempting to simply serve you."

In addition to these sources of power, one gains power by having information that she or he can control; from the people one knows and can call upon; and from a strong sense of self, knowing one's values, being self-confident, being able and willing to take risks, and standing up for that in which one believes. In order to increase one's power base, leaders and effective followers alike would do well to know themselves, develop a strong self-concept, develop and use good communication skills, establish support groups and networks, develop and show their expertise (i.e., market themselves), be willing to take risks, build coalitions, eliminate unnecessary dependence, understand "the system" and how it works, and be politically astute and active. Perhaps completing a tool like the "Power Perception Profile," developed by Hersey and Natemeyer (*http://www.ncsu.edu/csleps/leadership/eac301_word_documents/POWER_PERCEPTION_PROFILE.doc*), may help leaders and followers appreciate their sources of power and how effectively they use power.

In a very thoughtful book entitled, *The Power Tactics of Jesus Christ*, Haley (1989) summarized what he believed were the strategies Jesus used to realize his vision: He spoke whenever and wherever an audience would listen. He said what was unorthodox. He spoke openly about existing problems or injustices, consistently, publicly, and cleverly. He chose others to join in the "movement." He did not ask more of others than He was willing to give Himself. He articulated long-range plans. He used a flexible strategy, and He put His hope in the young, those who had not yet become entrenched in established ways. Through strategies such as these, Haley claimed, Jesus Christ came to be a powerful force for change.

EMPOWERING SELF AND OTHERS

As noted earlier, leaders engage in several tasks (Gardner, 1989) that help define them as leaders. Among those tasks are several that, in reality, can be thought of as means to empower oneself and one's followers. By *affirming values*, leaders help followers reflect on and perhaps challenge their values and the values of others. This helps followers become more powerful, as they come to know clearly what it is they believe and are willing to invest in. By *motivating followers*, leaders unlock or channel motives, promote positive attitudes, and encourage creativity, all of which empower followers to believe in themselves and take action. By striving to *achieve a workable unity*, leaders establish trust, cohesion and mutual tolerance, circumstances that empower followers to focus on the "big picture" and move out of their own "little corner of the world." *Explaining* helps followers understand the vision, why they are being asked to do certain things, and how they can and do contribute to achieving the group's goals. Followers are empowered by information and understanding. By *serving as a symbol*, a risk taker who acts as the group's source of unity, voice of anger, collective identity and source of hope, the leader helps followers seize the power that comes from debate, honest expression of feelings, and sharing in a struggle with others. Finally, through the process of *renewing*, both leaders and followers are empowered to breaking routines, habits, fixed attitudes, perceptions, assumptions, and unwritten rules, thereby allowing them to grow.

> *Each time a man stands up for an idea, or acts to improve the lot of others, or strikes out against injustice, he sends forth a tiny ripple of hope, and crossing each other from a million different centers of energy and daring, those ripples build a current that can sweep down the mightiest walls of oppression and resistance.*
>
> *Few are willing to brave the disapproval of their fellows, the censure of their colleagues, the wrath of their society. Moral courage is a rarer commodity than bravery in battle or greater intelligence. Yet it is the one essential, vital quality for those who seek to change a world that yields most painfully to change.* —Robert Kennedy

Gladwell (2000) notes that "there are exceptional people out there who are capable of starting epidemics" (p. 132). These are the "tempered radicals" (Meyerson, 2001) who "want to rock the boat, and [at the same time] stay in it" (p. xi). What underlies successful epidemics or revolutions "is a bedrock belief that change is possible [and] that people can radically transform their behavior or beliefs" (Gladwell, 2000, p. 258).

Followers can be helped to believe that change is possible, transform their behavior or beliefs, and start epidemics or revolutions, if leaders use the power they have to continually move the group toward the vision and to empower followers. Empowered followers do not materialize simply because a leader has acted to empower them. They can and do engage in activities that will enhance their followership skills.

STRATEGIES TO DEVELOP EFFECTIVE FOLLOWERSHIP SKILLS

Although there are many opportunities to assume the role of leader, each of us also will have countless opportunities to function as a follower (Fig. 3–5). We need to

FIGURE 3–5 · The follower role is quite common.

consciously develop the skills of followership and cultivate and appreciate that role so that we can draw on those skills to assume the mantle of leadership when that becomes necessary.

In a commentary on heroes and brave men, Barnum (1987) noted that "sometimes a field, any field, needs a hero or a bunch of heroes, an elite to set its course, to chart new lands, to brave new waters" (p. 5); the hero clears the way and "blazes the trail." Yet the only trails today's leaders can suggest, according to Barnum, "are slippery, fraught with rock slides, and inevitably lead up steep mountain sides" (p. 5), making it difficult for even the best of followers. Despite this challenge, however, in the contemporary world—and even more so in the future—the heroes may have the easier job and the followers the more difficult one.

Barnum asserted that "never before has the action of the masses had such potential to influence the direction of our profession" (1987, p. 5). Nurses who practice at the bedside demonstrate quality patient care, not the administrator who writes standards of care. It is the nurse working in the community who can influence local legislators with personalized human stories about the pain and suffering associated with polluted environments, lack of food, inadequate shelter, and poor prenatal care, not the statisticians who merely cite numbers and trends without providing a human dimension. The student experiencing the curriculum and the teacher/student relationships can best speak to the quality and effectiveness of the learning environment that exists in a school, not the faculty who design experiences but do not "live" them. In other words, followers have the most significant impact on the future of our profession and the world, an idea supported by Vaclav Havel, the dissident, poet, and ex-president of The Czech Republic who advocated solidarity in Communist Czechoslovakia and asserted and demonstrated that "followers hold significant power, even in totalitarian states, . . . if they act on it" (Kelley, 1992, p. 235).

If it is true that the future of our profession and the world will be most significantly affected by the actions of followers, then each of us needs to develop effective skills of followership. This notion has been expressed by many, (Chaleff, 1995, 1998; DiRienzo, 1994; Guidera & Gilmore, 1988; Kelley, 1992, 1998; Litzinger & Schaefer, 1984; Lundy, 1993; Meyerson, 2001; Pittman, Rosenbach, & Potter, 1998), but how can we develop such skills? According to Chaleff (1998, p. 89), "follower skills are learned informally, like street fighting," but they are, nevertheless, learned.

In her book on "paths to leadership," Andersen (1999) did not talk about followers or followership, per se. She and the various contributing authors talked about how students can chart a course toward assuming leadership positions in nursing. Inherent in those discussions was an implication that one develops as a leader by being an effective follower, a strategy Kelley (1992) refers to as "apprenticeship." Indeed, Aristotle, Plato, Homer, and Hegel, among others, insist that mastering followership is a necessary part of becoming an effective leader (Kelley, 1992; Rosenbach & Taylor, 1998).

Thus, one of the strategies suggested for nurses who aspire to effective followership and leadership is to apprentice yourself as a follower by assuming that role, thinking about what it means, reflecting on how you are contributing to your organization and the nursing profession by fulfilling that role, and *being the best you can be*. In addition, you would do well to study and implement many of the strategies that are suggested (later in this text and elsewhere) for developing leaders because those roles are so complementary. Among the strategies to help you be a more effective or exemplary follower are the following:

- Continue your education, both formal and informal. Knowledge is power and will serve you well as a follower.
- Be involved in your practice setting. Have a sense of ownership and stewardship; do not be merely a spectator.
- Take initiative. Take action without being told to do so.
- Be committed to something other than your own career development. Find your passion in life, and be passionate about what you do.
- Know your organization.
- Know your values and hold on to them.
- Set high standards. Others will model that.
- When they impede progress, be willing to "bend, circumvent, or break the rules to get things done" (Chaleff, 1995, p. 47).
- Be involved in professional organizations.
- Seek mentors or accept an offer of mentoring if it is made.
- Develop your professional networks—within and outside your organization —and use them.
- Accept a place at the table where decisions are made, or if such a place is not offered, create such a place for yourself. For example, agree to serve on a committee when invited to do so or volunteer to revise the admission data form if the one currently being used focuses too much on patient weaknesses and limitations and does not adequately address patient strengths and abilities.
- Feel free to criticize, but do not just complain and walk away. "Reflective backtalk increases a leader's ability to make good decisions" (Bennis, 2004, p. 2).
- Be proactive. Advocate and be a catalyst for change.
- Remain fully accountable for your actions.
- Share information rather than hoard it.
- Help colleagues grow and do their job well. Help them develop the skills of giving needed feedback.
- Be reflective.
- Have a sense of humor and laugh at your own mistakes.
- Develop positive relationships with colleagues, rely on each other, and be responsible to each other. Be a good team player.
- Continue to develop a wide array of skills in communication, assertiveness, clinical practice, decision-making, and writing.
- Analyze your performance by asking others for feedback and being honest in your own self-appraisal. Do you engage in gossip? Do you use language that suggests you are not as important as other people, or your ideas and suggestions are not as valuable as theirs? Do you allow yourself to be subservient? Are you cynical? Do you allow the leader or others to show disrespect for your coworkers' ideas or views? Are you willing to take risks? Are you destructive when you offer criticism?
- Contribute as an equal partner.

- Independently think up and champion new ideas.
- Try to solve difficult problems rather than expecting the leader to do it all.
- Figure out the steps needed for the group to achieve its goals, then be sure to be an integral part of those steps rather than on the periphery of "the action."
- Be cooperative with, rather than adversarial to, the leader.
- Appreciate the needs, goals, and constraints placed on the leader.
- Play devil's advocate. "Effective leaders reward dissent, as well as encourage it" (Bennis, 2004, p. 2).
- Give credit where it is due.
- Follow through on your commitments. Be credible.
- Know your job and do it well. Be competent, demonstrate your value to the group, and make a difference to the organization.
- Exercise a "courageous conscience . . . the ability to judge right from wrong and the fortitude to take affirmative steps toward what [you] believe is right" (Kelley, 1992, p. 168).
- Understand the importance of speaking out . . . and do it! "It is the good follower's obligation to share his or her best counsel with the person in charge. And silence—not dissent—is the one answer that leaders should refuse to accept" (Bennis, 2004, p. 2).
- Be enthusiastic and spread that enthusiasm to others.
- Know yourself, and be honest with yourself.
- Be comfortable with uncertainty and ambiguity. Resist the understandable fear of the unknown.
- Seek wise counsel.
- Speak up so others can benefit from your views. Speak the truth and be willing to "stand up, to stand out, to risk rejection, to initiate conflict" (Chaleff, 1995, p. 7).
- Present your position in a forthright manner. Develop excellence in communication by using a variety of channels.
- Develop self-confidence. Believe in and have faith in yourself.
- Remain calm. Do not be hostile.
- "Discover or create opportunities to fulfill [your] potential and maximize [your] value to the organization" (Chaleff, 1995, p. 6).
- Provide opportunities for the leader to talk about his or her vulnerabilities and concerns, as well as his or her strengths and vision.
- Help sacred cows be "gently led to pasture" (Chaleff, 1995, p. 89) so that all subjects are open to discussion and all options are possible. Do not discard what may seem like wild ideas before considering them carefully.
- Develop a record of successes.
- Do deep breathing or other relaxation exercises before having a conversation with an authority figure.
- Do not give in to peer pressure.
- Ask for feedback.
- Set personal goals and take responsibility to meet them.

- Stand up for and support your leader when he or she needs to make difficult decisions.
- Ask a great deal of the leader, but do not expect perfection from him or her.
- Express skepticism about ideas, proposals, and "pronouncements," but do so in a respectful way.
- "Learn the ropes," "pay your dues," and prove yourself in the follower role.
- Be dependable and reliable.
- Be creative.
- "Refuse to be used and abused" (Barron, 1998, p. 2).

It is obvious that there are many ways in which you can be an effective or exemplary follower. It also is obvious that it is only with concerted personal effort that you will develop the skills of effective followership. These "keys to effective followership" may be summarized in many ways, but the listing offered by Barron (1998, p. 2) seems to "say it all":

- Be a critical thinker, not a "yes" person.
- Be consistent and dependable.
- Be humble and patient.
- Be able to receive and offer constructive criticism.
- Be a tireless worker.
- Be a disciplined student of study and work (theory and practice).
- Be persistent and consistent at developing leadership (and followership) skills.
- Be a thinker!
- Be a thinker!!
- Be a thinker!!!

CONCLUSION

Followers have more power than they may realize. They confer the leadership role, and "the responsibility for making the leader-follower relationship work remains with the 'follower'" (Berg, 1998, p. 33). Indeed, followers can create a "conspiracy" (Bennis, 1989) that, although largely unconscious, can prevent leaders from leading, keeping them from "taking charge and making changes" (p. xii). "We are a nation of followers" (Kelley, 1992, p. 24), where "the spirit of American democracy elevates and celebrates the role of the follower" (p. 24). In such a society, the masses actually create history, and because "healthy followership is a conscious act of free will" (Chaleff, 1995, p.151), the masses allow certain individuals to exert leadership. Leaders, then, are accountable to followers, and followers play a significant role.

All of us are both leaders and followers, and most of us are followers more than we are leaders. That, however, is not anything for which we should apologize or anything about which we should feel badly. "Leaders cannot function without the eyes and ears and minds and hearts of followers" (DePree, 1992, p. 200), and they "only really accomplish something by permission of the followers" (p. 201). "The mark of a great leader is the development and growth of followers. The mark of a great follower is the growth of leaders" (Chaleff, 1995, p. 27). Therefore, instead of feeling insignificant in the role of follower, we should rejoice!

CRITICAL THINKING EXERCISES

What is appealing about being in the follower role? What is unattractive about being in that role?

_____

_____

Review the characteristics of effective followers. How would you describe yourself in the follower role? How effective have you been in that role?

_____

_____

Talk to your nursing colleagues about followership. What are their views on the concept? Was the concept ever addressed in their educational programs? Do they rate themselves as effective followers? How did they develop the abilities to be effective in that role? Whom do they identify as the most effective followers among their work group? What is the basis for that rating? Are these the same individuals they identify as leaders (or potential leaders) among the group?

_____

_____

How do your colleagues' opinions on followership and its development compare with your own views? How are nurses' views similar to or different from those outside health-care or those outside a predominantly female field?

_____

_____

Should we perhaps focus more on developing enlightened followers in nursing than on developing leaders all around us?

_____

_____

Read Chaleff's (1995, pp. 177–178) "Meditation on Followership." Are these principles by which you could live and that could guide your practice as a follower? This meditation may be something to review regularly as you implement your role as a professional nurse.

Meditation on Followership

I am a steward of this group and share responsibility for its success.
I am responsible for adhering to the highest values I can envision.
I am responsible for my successes and failures and for continuing to learn from them.
I am responsible for the attractive and unattractive parts of who I am.
I can empathize with others who are also imperfect.
As an adult, I can relate on a peer basis to other adults who are the group's formal leaders.
I can support leaders and counsel them, and receive support and counsel from them.
Our common purpose is our best guide.
I have the power to help leaders use their power wisely and effectively.
If leaders abuse power, I can help them change their behavior.
If I abuse power, I can learn from others and change my behavior.
If abusive leaders do not change their behavior, I can and will withdraw my support.
By staying true to my values, I can serve others well and fulfill my potential.
Thousands of courageous acts by followers can, one by one, improve the world.
Courage always exists in the present. What can I do today?

—*I. Chaleff*

_____

_____

Complete the following "Followership Style Test." What did you learn about yourself by taking this test? What did you learn about followership and the relationship between followers and leaders?

FOLLOWERSHIP STYLE TEST

This questionnaire includes statements about the type of boss you prefer. Imagine your-self to be in a subordinate position of some kind and use your responses to indicate your preference for the way in which a leader might relate with you.

The format includes a five-point scale: "Strongly Agree" (SA), "Agree" (A), "Mixed Feelings" (MF), "Disagree" (D), and "Strongly Disagree" (SD). Select one point on each scale and mark it as you read the 16 statements relating to followership.

	STATEMENT	SA	A	MF	D	SD
1.	I expect my job to be very explicitly outlined for me.	1	2	3	4	5
2.	When the boss says to do something, I do it. After all, he or she is the boss.	1	2	3	4	5
3.	Rigid rules and regulations usually cause me to become frustrated and inefficient.	5	4	3	2	1
4.	I am ultimately responsible for and capable of self-discipline based on my contacts with the people around me.	5	4	3	2	1
5.	My job should be made as short in duration as possible so that I can achieve efficiency through repetition.	1	2	3	4	5
6.	Within reasonable limits, I will try to accommodate requests from persons who are not my boss because these requests are typically in the best interests of the company anyway.	5	4	3	2	1
7.	When the boss tells me to do something that is the wrong thing to do, it is his or her fault, not mine, when I do it.	1	2	3	4	5
8.	It is up to my boss to provide a set of rules by which I can measure my performance.	1	2	3	4	5
9.	The boss is the boss. The fact of the promotion suggests that he or she has something on the ball.	1	2	3	4	5
10.	I accept orders only from my boss.	1	2	3	4	5
11.	I would prefer my boss to give me general objectives and guidelines then allow me to do the job my way.	5	4	3	2	1
12.	If I do something that is not right, it is my own fault, even if my boss told me to do it.	5	4	3	2	1
13.	I prefer jobs that are not repetitious, the kind of task that is new and different each time.	5	4	3	2	1
14.	My boss is in no way superior to me by virtue of positions. He or she does a different kind of job, one that includes a lot of managing and coordinating.	5	4	3	2	1
15.	I expect my boss to give me disciplinary guidelines.	1	2	3	4	5
16.	I prefer to tell my boss what I will, or at least should, be doing. I am ultimately responsible for my own work.	5	4	3	2	1

Scoring

Score your followership style by simply averaging the numbers for your answers to the individual items. For example, if you scored item number one "Strongly Agree," you will find the point value of "1" for that answer. To obtain your overall followership style, add all the numerical values associated with the 16 followership items and divide by 16. The resulting average is your followership style.

SCORE	DESCRIPTION	FOLLOWERSHIP STYLE
Less than 2.0	Very autocratic	Cannot function well without programs and procedures; needs feedback
2.0–2.4	Moderately autocratic	Needs solid structure and feedback but can also carry on independently
2.5–3.4	Mixed	Mixture of above and below
3.5–4.0	Moderately participative	Independent worker; does not need close supervision, just a bit of feedback
More than 4.0	Very democratic	Self-starter, likes a challenge and likes to try new things by himself or herself

Source: Adapted from Douglas, L. M. (1992). *The effective nurse leader and manager* (4th ed.) (pp. 25–28). St. Louis: Mosby.

References

Anderson, C. F. (1999). *Nursing student to nursing leader: The critical path to leadership development.* Albany, NY: Delmar.

Barnum, B. (1987). The need for heros [sic] and the need for brave men. *Courier (Newsletter of the Teachers College, Columbia University Nursing Education Alumni Association) 54,* 5.

Barron, C. (1998). *Dare to lead.* Retrieved January 26, 1998 from *www.dynamicleadership. com/leader.html*

Barwick, J. (2007). Following the leader and leading the followers. In J. F. Wergin (Ed.), *Leadership in place: How academic professionals can find their leadership voice* (pp. 88–99). Bolton, MA: Anker Publishing.

Bass, B. M. (1990). *Bass and Stogdill's handbook of leadership* (3rd ed.). New York: Free Press.

Bennis, W. (1989). *Why leaders can't lead. The unconscious conspiracy continues.* San Francisco: Jossey-Bass.

Bennis, W. (2004). Followership. Accessed October 7, 2004 from, *http://www. graphicarts.org/nalc/articles/follower/htm*

Bennis, W. (2006). The end of leadership: Exemplary leadership is impossible without full inclusion, initiatives, and cooperation of followers. In W. E. Rosenbach & R. L. Taylor (Eds.), *Contemporary issues in leadership* (6th ed.) (pp. 129–142). Boulder, CO: Westview Press.

Berg, D. N. (1998). Resurrecting the muse. Followership in organizations. In E. B. Klein, F. Gabelnick & P. Herr (Eds.), *The psychodynamics of leadership* (pp. 27–52). Madison, CT: Psychosocial Press.

Brown, B. (1980). Follow the leader. *Nursing Outlook, 28*(6), 357–359.

Chaleff, I. (1998). Learn the art of followership. In W. E. Rosenbach & R. L. Taylor (Eds.), *Contemporary issues in leadership* (4th ed.) (pp. 89–91). Boulder, CO: Westview Press.

Chaleff, I. (1995). *The courageous follower. Standing up to and for our leaders.* San Francisco: Berrett-Koehler.

Corona, D. (1986). Followership: The indispensable corollary to leadership. In E. C. Hein & M. J. Nicholson (Eds.), *Contemporary leadership behavior: Selected readings* (2nd ed.) (pp. 87–91). Boston: Little, Brown.

DePree, M. (1992). *Leadership jazz.* New York: Doubleday Currency.

DiCarlo, P. (2002). Followership, followers and following. Accessed October 7, 2004 from *http://www.it-analysis.com/article_pf.php?articleid=3314*

DiRienzo, S. M. (1994). A challenge to nursing: Promoting followers as well as leaders. *Holistic Nursing Practice 9*(1), 26–30.

Dreher, D. (1996). *The Tao of personal leadership.* New York: HarperBusiness.

French, J. P., Jr., & Raven, B. (1960). The bases of social power. In D. Cartwright & A. Zander (Eds.), *Group dynamics* (pp. 607–623). New York: Harper and Row.

Gardner, J. W. (1989). The tasks of leadership. In W. E. Rosenbach & R. L. Taylor (Eds.), *Contemporary issues in leadership* (2nd ed.) (pp. 24–33). Boulder, CO: Westview Press.

Gladwell, M. (2000). *The tipping point: How little things can make a big difference.* Boston: Little, Brown.

Goffee, R., & Jones, G. (2006). Followership: It's personal, too. In W. E. Rosenbach & R. L. Taylor (Eds.), *Contemporary issues in leadership* (6th ed.) (pp. 127–128). Boulder, CO: Westview Press.

Goldsmith, B. (2007). Finding the great leader within. *Association Executive* (January/February), 24–25.

Guidera, M. K., & Gilmore, C. (1988). In defense of followership. *American Journal of Nursing, 88* (7), 1017.

Haley, J. (1989). *The power tactics of Jesus Christ.* New York: W. W. Norton.

Joel, L. A. (1999). Life review of an ANA President: The path of leadership. In C.A. Andersen (Ed.), *Nursing student to nursing leader: The critical path to leadership development* (pp. 17–32). Albany, NY: Delmar.

Kelley, R. (1992). *The power of followership: How to create leaders people want to follow and followers who lead themselves.* New York: Doubleday Currency.

Kelley, R. E. (1998). In praise of followers. In W. E. Rosenbach & R. L. Taylor (Eds.), *Contemporary issues in leadership* (4th ed.) (pp. 96–106). Boulder, CO: Westview Press.

Kohn, L. T., Corrigan, J. M., & Donaldson, M. S. (Eds.). (2000). *To err is human: Building a safer health system.* Washington, DC: National Academy Press.

Kouzes, J. M., & Posner, B. Z. (1993). *Credibility: How leaders gain and lose it. Why people demand it.* San Francisco: Jossey-Bass.

Litzinger, W., & Schaefer, T. (1984). Leadership through followership. In W. E. Rosenbach & R. L. Taylor (Eds.), *Contemporary issues in leadership* (pp. 138–143). Boulder, CO: Westview Press.

Lundy, J. L. (1993). *Lead, follow, or get out of the way. Invaluable insights into leadership styles.* San Diego: Pfeiffer & Co.

Meyerson, D. E. (2001). *Tempered radicals: How people use difference to inspire change at work.* Boston: Harvard Business School Press.

O'Neil, E., & Coffman, J. (Eds.). (1998). *Strategies for the future of nursing: Changing roles, responsibilities, and employment patterns of registered nurses.* San Francisco: Jossey-Bass.

Pittman, T. S., Rosenbach, W. E., & Potter, E. H., III. (1998). Followers as partners: Taking the initiative for action. In W. E. Rosenbach & R. L. Taylor (Eds.), *Contemporary issues in leadership* (4th ed.) (pp. 107–120). Boulder, CO: Westview Press.

Porter-O'Grady, T. (1993). Of mythspinners and mapmakers: 21st century managers. *Nursing Management, 24*(4), 52–55.

Potter, E. H., III, & Rosenbach, W. E. (2006). Followers as partners: The spirit of leadership. In W.E. Rosenbach & R. L. Taylor (Eds.), *Contemporary issues in leadership* (6th ed.) (pp. 143–153). Boulder, CO: Westview Press.

Reed, M. (2004, August 26). Transformational servant leadership. Webinar sponsored by Encounter Collaborative.

Rocchiccioli, J. T., & Tilbury, M. S. (1998). *Clinical leadership in nursing.* Philadelphia: Saunders.

Rosenbach, W. E., & Taylor, R. L. (1998). Followership: The underappreciated dimension. In W. E. Rosenbach & R. L. Taylor (Eds.), *Contemporary issues in leadership* (4th ed.) (pp. 85–88). Boulder, CO: Westview Press.

Salacuse, J. (2005). *Leading leaders: How to manage smart, talented, rich, and powerful people.* Boston: AMACOM.

Staub, R. E., II. (1996). *The heart of leadership: 12 practices of courageous leaders.* Provo, UT: Executive Excellence Publishing.

Sullivan, T. J. (1998). *Collaboration: A health care imperative.* New York: McGraw-Hill.

Swansburg, R. C., & Swansburg, R. J. (1999). *Introductory management and leadership for nurses* (2nd ed.). Sudbury, MA: Jones & Bartlett.

Swansburg, R. C., & Swansburg, R. J. (2002). *Introductory management and leadership for nurses* (3rd ed.). Sudbury, MA: Jones & Bartlett.

Wheatley, M. J. (1999). *Leadership and the new science. Discovering order in a chaotic world* (2nd ed.). San Francisco: Berrett-Koehler.

Yoder-Wise, P. S. (2003). *Leading and managing in nursing* (3rd ed.). St. Louis: Mosby.

CHAPTER 4

Leadership as an Integral Component of a Professional Role

LEARNING OBJECTIVES
- Identify characteristics of transformational and transactional leaders.
- Compare and contrast the leader–follower relationship in a transformational environment and a transactional environment.
- Explain how transformational leadership generates growth in an individual, an organization, and a group.
- Describe how Maslow's hierarchy of needs relates to leadership development.
- Explain how leadership ability is enhanced by emotional intelligence.
- Explain how leadership is an integral component of being a nurse professional.

INTRODUCTION

Professional nurses can no longer think of themselves as "just nurses." Nurses are increasingly expected to provide leadership, whether they hold staff positions or are vice presidents, nurse practitioners, or nurse educators. Therefore, it is important for all professional nurses to be self-confident, have a high degree of self-esteem, and be visionary. (See Chapter 5 for a discussion of vision.) Individuals with these strengths will be able to exert leadership in making decisions, facilitate partnerships with patients and other healthcare workers, accomplish goals, and reach stated visions.

It also is important for nurses to be competent if they are to provide leadership. Maxwell (1999) described three types of competent people:

1. Competent to identify what needs to happen
2. Competent and able to make it happen
3. Competent to make something happen when it really matters

Nurse leaders know what needs to happen to achieve quality patient care and excellence in nursing education. Nurses who are just beginning their careers can be excellent leaders and make a great contribution to the profession while at the same time jump-starting their career. Just look at the Robert Wood Johnson Foundation's *Transforming Care at the Bedside* initiative, and it becomes apparent that staff nurses must lead (Institute for Healthcare Improvement, 2007). They have the skills to achieve these goals and know the time for such action is now.

When thinking about the leadership that is exercised in a nursing group or organization, it must be realized that every individual, not just the nurse manager or dean or committee chair, has the potential and the responsibility to assume the role of leader and work with others to fulfill the goals of the group/organization. The individual who happens to be in the appointed, authoritative role (e.g., the nurse manager) may or may not be the person who actually fulfills the role of the leader. As discussed earlier, effective followers have skills comparable to those of leaders, and the effectiveness of the leadership that any individual provides depends largely on the followers. Gardner (1990) said, "Leadership can be distributed among members, and the leader must recognize the needs of the followers, help them see how these needs can be met, and give them confidence that they can accomplish results through their efforts" (p. 149). So, leaders must be able to lead others as well as themselves. If there is a determined and powerful followership, leaders can be successful. Hence, as strong followers, effective nurses actually are exerting leadership, cognizant of the unique characteristics and talents of their veteran, baby boomer, X and Y generation colleagues (Hill, 2004).

It is common, however, for nurses to fail to be effective followers or leaders. Consider the following situations. Instead of acting as leaders or effective followers, nurses criticize their managers, the institution, the director, the physician, or other people occupying positions of leadership. Nurses blame other nurses, failing to collaborate with each other. Nurses fail to challenge the "orders" of a physician, fail to capitalize on their extensive knowledge or experience, or claim to be "only a nurse" when talking to a physician or a patient. These examples point to low self-esteem. If nurses are to increase their responsibility and if the profession is to survive and thrive, all nurses must exercise their leadership ability. Nurse leaders also need to be authentic leaders, that is, they need to "bring love, hope, relationship-centered principles and inspiration to the workplace every day and inspire excellence" (Kerfoot, 2006, p. 319). Authenticity can only be defined by others not by the nurse, and it is the perception of the staff that the leader is "real, sincere, and defined by honesty and integrity that means the leader is authentic" (Kerfoot, 2006, p. 319).

Individuals are not born leaders; rather, leaders emerge and continue to evolve as a result of experiences, purposeful self-development, and interactions with a variety of people. All nurses need to practice their leadership and encourage others to get involved, either as effective followers or as leaders. By creating a vision, strategizing how to accomplish the vision, seeking creative ways to implement change, and effectively leading or following in a collaborative manner, nurses exercise the leadership skills that will assist the entire healthcare team in accomplishing the goal of quality patient care. In other words, a more positive and passionate outlook must prevail in our work environments. Chang (2001) recommended we provide this by revitalizing our work environments so they are comfortable, engaging, inspiring, and prevent burnout.

TYPES OF LEADERSHIP

In a classic work that still has relevance (more than 30 years later,) Burns (1978) described two types of leadership that are used to make change and create new futures: transactional leadership and transformational leadership.

Transactional Leadership

Transactional leadership involves an exchange in which both the leader and the followers "get something." The leader gets the job completed or the goal achieved, and the followers get promotions, money, or other benefits. The focus of this type of leadership system is the accomplishment of a task, and it is the type often seen in healthcare organizations. Some even argue that nurses too often focus on tasks.

Transactional leaders focus on getting the job done and see task completion as the "bottom line." Zaleznik (1989) characterized transactional leaders as manipulative, detached, and inscrutable. Although there may be some type of "connection" between these leaders and their followers, this connection often is something other than a common purpose or a shared vision. With such a relationship, both leaders and followers may perceive their work only as a job, and not invest in it as a career. As such, this philosophical approach, as we have seen in all too many hospital settings, is limiting.

Transformational Leadership

In contrast, transformational leadership is a process in which "leaders and followers raise one another to higher levels of motivation and morality" (Burns, 1978, p. 20). This motivation energizes people to perform beyond expectations by creating a sense of ownership in reaching the vision. Bass (1985, pp. 62, 67) compared transformational leadership with inspirational leadership that arouses motivation of followers. He cited examples of transformational leadership from a Reserve Officers Training Corps (ROTC) study, including the following:

- Instilling pride in all
- Building morale through "pep talks"
- Acting as a positive role model
- Building the confidence of others through personal encouragement
- Complimenting individuals' performances and contributions as a way to instill pride in the group

Bass (1985) characterized transformational leaders as charismatic, able to instill motivation in others, and able to give individualized consideration. Burns (1978) described them as individuals who heighten followers' awareness of what must be done to accomplish the shared goal. Bennis and Nanus (1985, p. 3) defined transformational leaders as individuals who "commit people to action, who convert followers into leaders, and who convert leaders into agents of change."

> All great leaders have had one characteristic in common: it was the willingness to confront unequivocally the major anxiety of their people in their time. —*John Kenneth Gailbraith*

Several strategies have been identified (Bennis & Nanus, 1985) to assist leaders to be more transformational: attention through vision, meaning through communication, trust through positioning, and deployment of self through positive self-regard and optimism about a desired outcome. In other words, transformational leaders emphasize the importance of following a vision and assisting others to participate in making it a reality; they communicate their values and beliefs to others so that they can achieve a common meaning in their work and realize the vision toward which all are striving; they trust others, are honest, and act responsibly; and finally, they use their talents and expertise as a way to express their desire and commitment to a vision. If nurses are to be transformational leaders, they must follow their dreams, communicate in an articulate manner, be concerned with their own growth as well as the growth of their followers, establish trusting relationships, and identify their strengths and limitations. They also need to readily accept change and constantly seek new ways of doing things despite the risk (Bass, 1985).

Bass (1985) and Burns (1978) believed that transformational leaders have strong personal value systems, and by sharing these values, they are able to affect and even change followers' beliefs, even without needing to negotiate "what's in it for the follower." In essence, transformational leaders have a spirit that creates special leader–follower relationships and promotes individual and group growth. In fact, this spirit, this feeling of mutual involvement, is of greater significance than any isolated task accomplishment. This excitement about a vision or idea that is worthwhile attracts others to follow.

Transformational Leadership and Nursing Practice

An example of how transformational leadership impacts patient care through increased nurse job satisfaction is described by Allen and Vitale-Nolen (2005). The implementation of a new patient care delivery model, namely *Relationship Based Nursing Model*, at New Hampshire Hospital improved nurse job satisfaction significantly with a 14% increase (N = 70). By redefining nursing care that encourages empowerment and consideration of both professional and personal values, this hospital's nurse leadership group generated a change in how nurses made decisions and validated that it is the nurse "who knows what to do [and how] to choose how to do it" (p. 281). Simply put, this creates an empowered environment "where nurses feel they make a difference" (p. 277).

Sashkin and Sashkin (2003) demonstrated in their research that many aspects of transformational leadership can be developed. Being able to recognize our colleagues' feelings, motivate others, and manage one's emotions well in our relationships serves to foster an environment that facilitates transformational leadership. For example, with the multi-faceted problems healthcare organizations face today, there are numerous crises that demand the entire staff, ranging from the maintenance crew to the chief executive officer, to be able to communicate to the public in a positive and non-threatening manner. How to convey this message using appropriate wording and emotion with the ever-changing technology of communications is part of everyone's responsibility (Fearn-Banks, 2007).

EMOTIONAL INTELLIGENCE

Goleman (1998) suggested that one of the most important attributes of leadership is emotional intelligence, which is quite different from one's intelligence quotient (IQ). He defined emotional intelligence as a group of competencies that influence our ability to respond to others and manage our own feelings. His research indicates that emotional intelligence is nearly twice as significant as IQ in becoming a leader. People are born with certain cognitive abilities, or IQ, and that is not likely to change dramatically throughout one's life, but emotional intelligence is something one can acquire. It is essential for nurses to realize the power they have in making positive change on their units, in their agencies, and in the health policy arena. Currently, in America, nurses are perceived to be among the most honest workers. This, coupled

Emotional Intelligence/Patient Care Case Study

The following is a case study about how emotionally intelligent nurses can impact their job satisfaction as well as their patients' care. Cynthia came from one of the urban acute trauma centers to the community hospital to be the nurse manager of the inpatient Orthopedic Unit and outpatient Orthopedic Center. She decided to work as a staff nurse one day/week on the unit and one-half day in the outpatient Orthopedic Surgery and Rehabilitation Center. She quickly established rapport with the patients, staff, and physicians in both areas. Her clinical competency with new orthopedic technology as well as her charismatic manner of leadership was highly respected by the staff. She collaborated with the physicians and members of the units' staff to determine if the hospital could purchase more equipment in order to expand their services. This was determined to be a definite "yes." Data showed that most orthopedic patients were waiting up to 3 months for surgery, so some were going to other hospitals far from their homes. The units in both the hospital and outpatient clinics were expanded for surgical procedures, and additional staff was hired to manage the workload. Cynthia felt it would be more cost effective and satisfying for the nurses and technicians in each area to be able to rotate [similar to the physicians] through the different settings with the new expansion. She set up a Committee to explore this option. The Committee, under her leadership, found that 90% of the nurses, assistants, and technicians were supportive of the rotations, though 10% preferred to stay in their current position. The units had a meeting to discuss these findings, and it was unanimously decided that the 10% not desiring to rotate would not have to rotate. The nurses were quite excited about the idea of having a new and expanded scope of practice. Cynthia assisted the Committee in setting up in-services, orientations, and precepting for each individual, so they would be prepared for this rotating unit schedule. Nurses volunteered to present the in-services and orientations, as well as to precept for each other. Once the scheduling was set up and piloted, the staff was able to anticipate potential problems and deal with them. Schedules were tweaked, and staff worked in a cohesive way. One year later, job and patient satisfaction were at the highest ever obtained. Length of stay was the lowest ever measured, and the cost of managing the units was down. Nurses were excited to learn new aspects of orthopedics and were joining the Orthopedic Nursing Society, becoming certified by the American Nursing Credentialing Center, attending conferences and reporting findings back, and conducting two evidence-based practice studies. The nurse manager asked for feedback from her staff every six months and found that the staff was overwhelmingly supportive of her leadership. Using the skills of emotional intelligence, Cynthia was successful in turning her unit into a cost generating unit where staff morale and retention increased.

with having high emotional intelligence, puts nurses in a position to impact the status quo.

Goleman, Boyatzis and McKee (2002) recommended that leaders need the following skills: self-awareness, self-regulation, motivation, empathy, and social skills. It is through using these skills that all leaders can reach out and touch or inspire others by effecting change, being creative, articulating visions, helping visions become reality, managing conflict, taking risks, networking, and adapting to new initiatives. Nurse leaders can use their emotional intelligence to create productive work environments for their units (Vitello-Ciccui, 2003). Leaders can maximize their successes as well as facilitate others' achievements by fostering an environment more conducive to using emotional intelligence, such as by sponsoring staff recognition days, publishing accomplishments in a unit/agency newsletter, and having peer-evaluated employee-of-the-month designations. Increasing our self-awareness, which is an important aspect of emotional intelligence, will most likely help build high self–esteem.

SELF-ESTEEM AND LEADERSHIP IMAGE

Barker, Sullivan, and Emery (2006) believed the most significant tool for transformational leaders to be effective is oneself, particularly one's self-awareness, self-development and one's trust of followers. They called this positive self-regard, which is very similar to how Bennis and Nanus (1985) described transformational leaders. Barker, Sullivan, and Emery (2006) and Burns (1978) suggested that Maslow's (1970) concept of self-esteem would be enhanced, if it included the concept of positive self-regard. Self-esteem includes the need for achievement, mastery, competence, confidence, independence, and freedom to act. Satisfying one's self-esteem needs tends to result in higher self-confidence and eventually self-actualization (Maslow, 1998). These abilities are congruent with those who define transformational leaders and effective followers, and since individuals who have high self-esteem are able to develop and grow, followers can become leaders.

Each of us must be self-motivated to change or improve our personal and professional lives. Individuals who are not motivated to change will most likely maintain the status quo and fail to provide leadership to or facilitate others' growth. However, one

---

BOX 4-1 **Expect Success Through Self-Confidence, Not Entitlement**

"One young lady had listed everything she had done to get into the finals, all of her exercising, her nutritional plans, her workouts, all of the sweat and pain and exertion and self-denial that she had gone through, and then she had written, 'DESERVE a place on the Olympic team!' I [as her coach] had to take her aside and give her a short lecture about that kind of thinking.

"Look, I said. You don't deserve squat. Every other person in these trials has done exactly what you have done—they have exercised, they have sweated, they have gone through pain, they have given up other pleasures, they are just as deserving as you are. Saying that you deserve something special puts you in the role of potential victim, so that you can later say, 'Poor me, life has failed me.'

"I told her, you can say I EXPECT to earn a place on the Olympic team. That's okay, that's an expression of self-confidence, a stance from where you can perform better because you expect to be among the best, but let's not have any more of these victimizing statements."

should not expect success simply because one feels that he or she has worked very hard. A good example of this entitlement issue is depicted in the story (see Box 4–1) of an aspiring pre-Olympian who would not likely be a transformational leader to her teammates because she is so self-oriented (Campbell, 1996, p. 9).

Many nurses have the attitude that they deserve more simply because they have seniority or have "paid their dues." When they don't get more, they allow themselves to be victims of the system. Things do not change just because people think they deserve special favors (i.e., treatment that ignores system constraints); this only propagates more unhappiness and victimization for the nurse. Kouzes and Posner (1995) note that the unprecedented instability in today's world calls for strong leadership. They recommend that leaders engage in practices that transform followers and help realize visionary goals such as the following:

- Challenge the status quo.
- Inspire a shared vision.
- Enable others to act, rather than to react.
- Be role models.
- Encourage the heart.

The first four practices are self-explanatory. The last practice, "encouraging the heart," highlights the importance of leaders caring deeply about the vision and working hard to accomplish it. It also suggests that people who perform well, will be self-satisfied. Kouzes and Posner recommended that "leaders celebrate accomplishments," making others "feel like hero[es]" (1995, p. 318). In order to do this, individuals need to feel good about themselves. Nurses have been "controlled by forces outside themselves that had greater prestige, power, and status" (Roberts, 1983, p. 21) and we have, in essence, allowed ourselves to be exploited. Therefore, it is crucial that we enhance our initiative, self-esteem, assertiveness, and positive self-regard if we are to provide leadership in and advance our profession.

WOULD-BE LEADERS BECOME LEADERS

Nurses need to reinvent themselves, much as others have done. Bennis (1993) explained the process of reinventing himself "to avoid accepting roles [which he] was brought up to play" (p. xv). He further describes the significance of being able to invent and reinvent himself so that he would not have to be "content with borrowed postures, secondhand ideas, [or] fitting in instead of standing out" (p. xv). His warning not to accept stereotypical perceptions offers a lesson for nurses and non-nurses alike: Do not accept stereotypes of nursing. By reinventing oneself, we "do not accept the roles we were brought up to play" (Bennis, 1993, p. 2). If nurses reinvented themselves, focused on larger issues rather than merely the tasks of the day, refused to operate with tunnel vision, refused to act as "passive followers," and refused to remain in organizational positions that are less powerful (Kirchbaum, 1997, p. 12), ours would be a very different world! Another strategy is to use a more global perspective of connecting with others who are pursuing new initiatives, experiencing similar problems, or have resources that we can share with other organizations. Chayko (2002) shares multiple strategies for forming social bonds and community networks in her book, *Connecting: How We Form Social Bonds and Communities in the Internet Age*.

It is imperative to appreciate that nursing complements, but is not subservient to, other healthcare providers, and this perspective develops as one learns to be a nurse. In fact, Kirchbaum (1997) suggested that "nurse educators include in their nursing leadership and management course the idea of helping students realize their knowledge—that personal power, those abilities they possess which contribute to solving a problem or accomplishing their goals" (p.12)—is significant to the provision of high-quality care. It is imperative, therefore, that nurse educators foster leadership in their students, help students integrate leadership as an integral component of their role, and focus as much on the development of leadership skills as on the acquisition of clinical skills. Development of leadership skills must be a part of both the student's professional and personal journey in life. These skills need to be introduced literally from birth and reinforced by family, friends, and the community as well as the individual's school long before post-secondary education. Bolman and Deal (2001) described one such journey of an adult as he acquired the ability to lead with heart.

LEADERSHIP AS AN INTEGRAL COMPONENT OF EACH NURSE'S ROLE

Nurses are increasingly expected to assume the roles of advocate, teacher, caregiver, disseminator of knowledge, manager, contributor to public health policy development, and leader. Nurses are also expected to be heavily involved in partnering with other nurses and members of other healthcare disciplines to achieve quality patient care. Nurses, therefore, are expected to play a major role in evoking change in healthcare and ensuring their significant role in the restructured system of managed care.

Nurses must acquire principle-centered leadership to be effective in the new healthcare system. Principle-centered leadership involves "keeping promises, developing virtues, changing bad habits, being faithful to vows, exercising courage, and being genuinely considerate of others" (Covey, 1991, p. 18). These principles are similar to compasses in that they always point the way and keep us from becoming lost amid conflicting ideas and values. Covey (1991) says principles constantly apply and they surface in the form of "ideas, norms, values, and teachings which uplift, fulfill, empower, and inspire people" (p. 19). Characteristics that exemplify principle-centered leaders include continually learning, having a service orientation, having positive energy, believing in others, leading a balanced life, viewing life as an adventure, being synergistic, and having the ability to self-renew.

Leaders must also possess exceptional communication skills. Nurses, therefore, must be consistent, assertive, and knowledgeable speakers about their role, the state of the healthcare system, and their patients' care. Likewise, nurses would be more effective leaders if they possessed sophisticated interpersonal relationship skills to use with patients, families, communities, other healthcare providers, and the public.

Credibility is another important characteristic that admired leaders possess. Kouzes and Posner (1993, p. 50) studied people's reasons for respecting, trusting, and being willing to be influenced by others and found the following behaviors as indicative of credibility: supporting, having the courage to do the right thing, challenging, developing and acting as a mentor to others, listening, celebrating good work, following through on commitments, trusting others, empowering others, making time for people, sharing the vision, opening doors, overcoming personal hardships, admitting mistakes, advising others, solving problems creatively, and teaching well. These behaviors reflect the characteristics of a credible, transformational leader. The four components that correlated highest with being credible included honesty, competency, inspiration, and being forward-looking (Kouzes & Posner, 1993).

> *To achieve all that is possible, we must attempt the impossible . . . to be as much as we can be, we must dream of being more.* —Gale Baker Stanton

Nurses must be morally fit leaders, capable of using good ethical judgment in making decisions about delivering quality care to all patients. They must be patient advocates and representatives of their patients' needs. Each has obligations of promoting ethical leadership, composed of communication, quality, and collaboration (Rhode, 2006). Today's corporate scandals emphasize the need for nurses to lead ethically and morally.

Taking a risk to try something new, taking time to dream and imagine how one could make a difference, joining a professional organization and becoming actively involved, and taking courses for personal gain (e.g., public speaking) or to complete a degree or certificate, are all activities that nurses should consider as part of their self-renewal. By self-evaluating or using peer evaluation effectively, one can identify strengths and weaknesses, nurture one's strengths, and either work on or work around one's limitations. Nurses also need to become comfortable with "learn[ing] to learn while doing" (Margerison & Kakabadse, 1984, p. 24), rather than thinking we must be competent in everything we undertake, therefore often refusing promotions or transfers to other areas of practice because we feel it is safer to maintain what we already do "best." Leaders take risks.

As leaders in the healthcare arena today, nurses must embody the qualities mentioned here for nursing services to be accessible to patients, for nurses to be involved in multidisciplinary collaboration, and for nursing care to be identified as the reason for positive and cost-effective patient outcomes. Nurses can and must be leaders.

CONCLUSION

One does not have to be in nursing management to be a "true" nursing leader, so there are unlimited opportunities for nurses to exercise leadership. For many, that may require much self-reflection and reinvention. As Bennis (1993, p. 1) recommended, "people who cannot reinvent themselves must be content with borrowed postures, secondhand ideas, and fitting in instead of standing out."

Nurses are increasingly "standing out" and providing leadership as they begin new roles in promoting health in inner-city homeless centers, school-based health clinics, or taking healthcare vans to the most needy of people. Nurses are starting satellite outpatient dialysis and chemotherapy centers, cardiac rehabilitation centers, and preoperative learning clinics to assist people in restoring their health. Nurses in acute care areas are developing new nurse-driven protocols; collaborating with other healthcare disciplines in creating critical pathways that focus patient care on meeting outcomes; and participating in teaching smoking cessation, cholesterol lowering, and alternative nonpharmacological programs.

Many nursing leaders are making a difference in patient outcomes and using their leadership potential to meet their own expectations of self. We need more nurses like this. Nursing educators must revise curricula to provide students with opportunities to practice leadership as well as clinical roles. Nurse administrators need to create environments that encourage and support open dialogue, peer feedback, innovation, and change. Nurses tneed to mentor each other and call upon the strengths of one another, much like geese who fly in a "V" formation (see Box 4–2). When each nurse sees leadership as an integral component of her or his professional role, we will be able to transform healthcare.

BOX 4-2 **Learning Lessons from Geese**

Although we may know that geese fly in a "V" formation, what we may not know is that as each bird flaps its wings, it creates an uplift for the bird following. By flying in formation, the whole flock adds 71% more to the flying range than if each bird flew alone.

A second fact about geese is that when the lead goose gets tired, it moves back into the formation and another goose flies the point position.

Third, if a goose falls out of the formation, it feels the drag and resistance of trying to fly alone and quickly gets back into formation to take advantage of the power of the bird it follows.

What are the lessons here for leadership? First, leadership must be shared. We all must take our turn doing the work that will help our profession evolve, our organizations grow, and ourselves continue to develop. Second, every member of the group has the potential to "fly the point position" and serve as the leader; we should not limit our expectations of the potential within each of us. Finally, the work we do can stimulate and excite others in our group to also perform better and achieve a level of excellence perhaps previously unexpected. There is much we can learn about leaders and leadership from geese. We need only to pay attention and be open to new ideas, perspectives, and possibilities.

CRITICAL THINKING EXERCISES

Describe how you could reinvent yourself, personally and professionally, so as not to merely "live the status quo."

_____

_____

How would you describe individuals you think of as leaders? Individuals you do not consider to be leaders? What are some of the differences between these two groups of individuals in terms of a "leadership image?"

_____

_____

How would you describe the image you convey? Look at the way you dress, things you have written, presentations you have made, your participation on committees or in class, and so on. Is this the image you want to convey? If not, what aspects are unsatisfactory to you, and how could you change them?

_____

_____

Watch the film _Jerry McGuire_, and describe how the leaders have a sense of moral courage and the desire to speak up when something is not right. List some of the issues that you feel were "not right" and suggest leadership behaviors that you would use to do things "right."

_____

_____

Compare the "leadership image" of nurses in various roles: staff nurse, advanced practice nurse, nurse educator, nursing service administrator, and so on. How are they alike? How are they different? What kinds of things can a nurse do to convey a strong image?

_____

_____

What can aspiring nurse leaders do to overcome negative stereotypes of nurses and nursing, create a genuinely positive leadership image, and project that image to achieve desired goals?

_____

_____

Read Bolman & Deal's _Leading with Soul: An Uncommon Journey of Spirit_ (2001) and determine where you are on your journey of leadership.

_____

_____

References
_____

Allen, D., & Vitale-Nolen, R. (2005). Patient care delivery model improves nurse job satisfaction. *The Journal of Continuing Education in Nursing, 36*(6), 277–282.

Barker, A., Sullivan, D., & Emery, M. (2006). *Leadership competencies for clinical managers: The renaissance of transformational leadership.* Sudbury, MA: Jones and Bartlett Publishers.

Bass, B. (1985). *Leadership and performance beyond expectations.* New York: Macmillan.

Bennis, W. (1993). *An invented life: Reflections on leadership and change.* Reading, MA: Addison-Wesley.

Bennis, W., & Nanus, B. (1985). *Leadership: The strategies for taking charge.* New York: Harper & Row.

Bolman, L., & Deal, T. (2001). *Leading with soul: An uncommon journey of spirit* (2nd ed.). San Francisco: Jossey-Bass.

Burns, J. (1978). *Leadership.* New York: Harper & Row.

Campbell, D. (1996). Inklings. *Issues & Observations, 16*(1), 9.

Chayko, M. (2002). *Connecting: How we form social bonds and communities in the internet age.* Albany, NY: State University of New York.

Chang, R. (2001). *The passion plan at work.* San Francisco: Jossey-Bass.

Covey, S. (1991). *Principle-centered leadership.* New York: Summit Books.

Covey, S. (1989). *Seven habits of highly effective people: Conveying a leadership image.* New York: Fireside.

Covey, S. (2006). *The 8th habit: From effectiveness to greatness.* New York: Running Press Book Publishers.

Davis, C. (1991). Dress for success. *Nursing Spectrum*, March 25, 1991.

Fearn-Banks, K. (2007). *Crisis communications: A casebook approach* (3rd ed.). Mahwah, NJ: Lawrence Erlbaum Associates, Publishers.

Gardner, J. (1990). *On leadership.* New York: Free Press.

Goleman, D. (1998). *Working with emotional intelligence.* New York: Bantam Books.

Goleman, D., Boyatzis, R., & McKee, A. (2002). *Primal leadership: Realizing the power of emotional intelligence.* Boston: Harvard Business School Press.

Hill, K. (2004). Learn what motivates veterans, baby boomers, generation X and Y employees. *Nursing Management, 35*(1), 32–35.

Institute for Healthcare Improvement (IHI). (2007). *Transforming care at the bedside.* Retrieved July 22, 2007 from, *www.ihi.org.NR/rdonlyres*

Kerfoot, K. (2006). Authentic leadership. *MEDSURG Nursing, 15*(5), 319–320.

Kirchbaum, K. (1997). Preparing students for leadership in practice. *Creative Nursing, 3*(2), 12–14.

Kouzes, J., & Posner, B. (1993). *Credibility: How leaders gain and lose it, why people demand it*. San Francisco: Jossey-Bass.

Kouzes, J., & Posner, B. (1995). *The leadership challenge: How to keep getting extraordinary things done in organizations* (2nd ed.). San Francisco: Jossey-Bass.

Margerison, C., & Kakabadse, A. (1984). *How American chief executives succeed*. New York: American Management Association.

Maslow, A. (1970). *Motivation and personality* (2nd ed.). New York: Harper & Row.

Maslow, A. (1998). *Maslow on management*. New York: John Wiley.

Maxwell, J. (1999). *The 21 indispensable qualities of a leader: Becoming the person others will want to follow*. Nashville, TN: Thomas Nelson.

Rhode, D. (Ed.). (2006). *Moral leadership: The theory and practice of power, judgment, and policy*. San Francisco: Jossey-Bass.

Roberts, S. (1983). Oppressed group behavior: Implications for nursing. *Advances in Nursing Science, 5*(4), 21–30.

Sashkin, M., & Sashkin, M. (2003). *Leadership that matters: The critical factors for making a difference in people's lives and organizations' success*. San Francisco: Berrett-Koehler.

Vitello-Cicciu, J. (2003). Emotional intelligence. *Nursing Management, 34*(10), 29–32.

Zaleznik, A. (1989). *The managerial mystique: Restoring leadership in business*. New York: Harper & Row.

CHAPTER 5
Vision and Creativity

LEARNING OBJECTIVES
- Define the concept of vision as it relates to leadership.
- Describe how a nurse leader or follower can facilitate the identification, articulation, and communication of a personal vision.
- Identify strategies that would be effective in making one's personal vision become a reality.
- Formulate a personal vision for the profession or one's particular area of practice.
- Identify characteristics of nursing and non-nursing leaders who are viewed as visionary.
- Describe characteristics of creative persons, processes, and environments.
- Project potential outcomes of using creativity as a nurse leader or follower.
- Identify how the new science of leadership fosters creativity in order to improve leadership and followership.
- Examine how the incorporation of vision and creativity into one's professional role can help vitalize and energize a nurse.

INTRODUCTION

One of the most significant characteristics of a leader is to have a vision of a "better world." We use many words such as "vision," "impact," "empowerment," and "facilitation" in everyday conversation. The time has come to stop repeating the words and begin to take action.

Having a vision, as well as being able to energize followers to join in the effort of making that vision a reality, involves credibility, communication skills, an ability to maintain momentum, and creativity. Nurses typically are skilled in communication, have high energy levels, and are seen as credible. They often do not think of themselves as creative and have difficulty sustaining and capitalizing on the momentum of a group. The mere idea of being creative may seem foreign to nurses who are accustomed to following fairly strict protocols for delivering patient care. In addition, the expectation that nurses have and can articulate a vision also may seem unusual if one has been socialized to expect that only the chief nursing officer (CNO) or vice president has the right or responsibility to "have" a vision. Being able to incorporate a new philosophy of leadership into one's professional role, accepting responsibility for articulating a vision, and allowing oneself to be creative are all essential.

Leaders do many extraordinary things, but one of the greatest contributions they make is having a focus or a purpose that emerges from their knowledge and experience, their emotional intelligence (see Chapter 4), as well as their passion. This purpose then underpins their idea of what would facilitate the work of the group in question. There are three major aspects of visionary leadership: the construction of the vision to encompass the image of an organization or group, the development of a set of strategies that make the vision a driving force for the organization or group, and the ability to communicate the vision and engage every member of the organization or group towards making it become a reality (Sashkin, 1989). In order to lead, one must have a vision (Bennis, 1994).

THE CONCEPT OF VISION
What Is Vision?

Visions are dreams or ideas that are "specific enough to provide guidance to people yet vague enough to encourage initiative and to remain relevant under a variety of conditions" (Kotter, 1990, p. 36). A vision is also an image of where the organization or group wants to be in the future (Conger, 1989). A vision is different from a goal because it is broad and it does not focus on a "greater return on assets or increased market share or introduction of a new product" (Conger, 1989, p. 38). Kouzes and Posner (1993) studied 90 leaders in large organizations and found vision to be identified as a key strategy for their success. Some of the participants described a vision as "a purpose, mission, legacy, dream, goal, calling, [or] personal agenda" (p. 94). Conger (1989) believes that most visions can be categorized into one of four types (Fig. 5-1): those with an external orientation (e.g., a marketing innovation), those with an internal orientation (e.g., a transformation of the organization's mission), those that are narrow in focus, and those that are more broadly focused.

Obviously, a vision overlaps a variety of ideas and values in an organization or group. It may begin with an internal orientation and a narrow perspective, then grow into a more external direction with a broader perspective. In nursing, critical pathways may be a step in realizing the vision to "refocus care to the patient." For example, a nursing unit might begin by developing or implementing critical pathways for a few classic diagnostic-related groups (DRGs). As this idea takes hold among nurses, physicians, and other healthcare providers, word about the positive patient outcomes and cost-effective results of using the critical paths spreads to other departments in the organization (e.g., accounting, human resources, supplies,

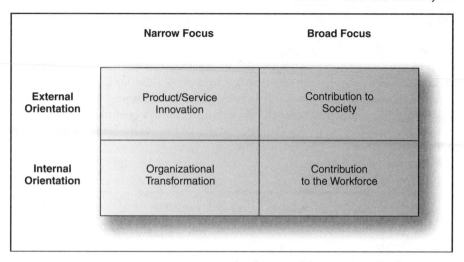

	Narrow Focus	**Broad Focus**
External Orientation	Product/Service Innovation	Contribution to Society
Internal Orientation	Organizational Transformation	Contribution to the Workforce

FIGURE 5-1 • A typology of visions. (Source: Conger, J. [1989] *The charismatic leader: Behind the mystique of exceptional leadership* [p. 44]. San Francisco: Jossey-Bass.)

staffing). Consumer representatives who had served on the committees to institute the redesign start sharing outcomes outside of the hospital, and soon there is likely to be more external community and consumer interest.

WHY HAVE A VISION?

One can have both personal and professional visions. Personal vision gives one a purpose in life, and professional vision helps one accomplish work ideas and the mission of an organization, group, or profession. The term co-missioning, created by Covey (2004), merges an individual's personal goals and the organization's vision. He describes this process as "the key to unleashing the power of the workforce" (p. 224). Co-missioning is defined as a way of linking mission and vision of a workplace so there are similarities with the employee's needs.

One must be able to identify opportunities to clarify one's vision and act on incorporating new strategies that would facilitate implementation of the vision. One also must be cognizant of the potential for "roadblocks" that may interfere with the vision becoming a reality, although roadblocks may, in the long run, actually assist in mobilizing people to change and accept a new plan or vision.

For example, the advanced practice nurses (APNs) at a new inner-city nurse-run clinic felt "blocked" by their medical director, who insisted that all new prescription orders be cosigned by a physician before the medication could be dispensed. Concurrently, the clinic administrator was negotiating with the director of the adjacent detention center regarding servicing the inmates. One of the detention center's primary needs was immediate service, including prescriptions for a very transient, mobile clientele who might be at the jail for only 1 to 2 hours per day. A contract with the detention center would generate a large amount of work and a positive image for the clinic; however, this agreement could not be made if the APNs could not independently dispense medications. The roadblock put up by the medical director (e.g., not allowing nurse practitioners to autonomously prescribe new medications) was overturned. The medical director attended a meeting to discuss the role of the APNs and the state's APN practice act. This meeting resulted in a better understanding of the APN role overall and an expanded mission for the nurse practitioner–run clinic, outcomes that never would have been achieved had it not been for the road-block regarding autonomous prescription writing. Thus, it is important for each nurse to think positively, speak in possibilities, and not give up. Stoltz (2000) defined such thinkers as "possibility leaders" who trigger a spark of possibility for others and stimulate change and reform.

> *The secret of leadership is . . . far-sightedness: gazing beyond the visible to the potential on the horizon.* —*J. Donald Walters*

Actualizing a Vision

Many leaders have demonstrated the importance of being flexible or being able to accept some unforeseen change in plans in order to actualize one's vision. When Bill Gates and Paul Allen founded Microsoft Corporation in 1975, their vision was to have a computer in every home, office, and school. Gates was a college student at the time, but he was able to visualize a new role for computers in our personal lives. He took a leave from his undergraduate program at Harvard to follow his dream, and he took risks, used his creative talent, convinced others, and kept pursuing his dream. Today, Gates is in his early 40s, and his company is the leading worldwide provider of person-al computer software with revenues of $11 billion annually. If he had not left school and risked going out on his own with Paul Allen, Bill Gates may have never actualized his dream, and computers would not have as dramatically changed our world as we have witnessed in recent years. Such is the power of dreams—of visions (Manes & Andrews, 1993).

Mother Teresa, winner of a Nobel Peace Prize in 1979, founded the Missionaries of Charity in Calcutta, India. She had to make a difficult decision to leave the order of nuns to which she belonged at the time in order to follow her vision—"helping the poorest of the poor while living among them" (LeJoly, 1983, p. 26). Mother Teresa worked from morning to night helping the poor and guiding the nuns who joined her to fulfill her vision. She was not satisfied with her purpose on earth as a nun in her original order, which felt like the status quo for her, so she took risks, used her creative talent, convinced others, and kept pursuing her dream, even without any funding. Mother Teresa founded a whole new order of sisters, provid-ed exquisite care to the world's poor, and made the world more conscious of the needs of millions of our fellow human beings. Such is the power of dreams—of visions.

Kouzes and Posner (1993) describe leaders as pioneers—people who are able and willing to "reach for the sky," people who are able to recognize a great idea, and

Vision without action is merely a dream. Action without vision passes the time. Vision and action can change the world. —Joel Barker

people who make change. Parse (1997) says a leader is "one who guides by blazing a path" (p. 109). She states that the path is a vision that offers something to others and that they can choose to follow or not. Many (Conger, 1989; Kotter, 1990; Porter-O'Grady & Wilson, 1995) believe that a leader's most significant function is to produce a change that cannot actually be identified as it transpires step-by-step but is more of a feeling that people grab onto, attempt to implement, and then share serendipitously! This perspective is most congruent with the new leadership, which suggests it would be nonproductive to be too orderly and attempt to implement a vision in a step-by-step fashion, as it is unlikely that no change would occur with such a linear approach.

Porter-O'Grady and Wilson (1995) believe the pace of change in and the advancement of an organization or group are strongly correlated to the underlying vision that guides it. Although these authors hesitate to recommend short-term goal setting because they are proponents of the new science of leadership, they do advocate that managers become leaders and break down the barriers of the bureaucratic organizational structure of which we are all so much a part. Perhaps then, and only then, will leaders and followers be successful in owning a vision that does not suggest a lockstep approach to achievement, but rather one that is open to possibilities and creative decision-making. Conger (1989) suggested that one positive advantage of having a vision is that it brings people a "sense of contribution to themselves, to an industry, or to a society," and "draws workers together as a team" (p. 43). To share the same vision, the leader must inspire followers, and the leader must value the followers' contributions (Kotter, 1990). Recognition for an extraordinary job in the form of an award, public announcement, or financial reimbursement might assist the follower to connect better to the overall vision.

An excellent example of a leader who had a dream, motivated others, and made followers feel as if they owned the dream was Dr. Martin Luther King, Jr. His "I Have a Dream" speech, delivered on August 28, 1963, at the Lincoln Memorial in Washington, DC, is a testament to the power of a vision and how it can energize people toward action. *(http://www.mecca.org/~crights/dream.html)*.

Dr. King's dream was clearly articulated, and the way he conveyed his vision showed his passion and enthusiasm and the extent to which it came from and reflected his inner being. Whether we work in administration; teaching; or clinical roles in schools, homes, hospitals, or clinics—or if we are students—each of us has a reason for why we became a nurse. That reason may have been to help others, to champion the "underdog," to care for others in need, or to develop healthcare programs for all. Perhaps some of us need to reflect on our original dream and think about how what we are currently doing relates to why we wanted to be nurses in the first place. It is possible that our original idea of why we chose to enter nursing is still important and drives us to enjoy our present work; but it also is possible that we are stuck in a "dead end" or a "rut" and feel that we are not fulfilled. For those of us who get up day after day without thinking about why we do what we do, it may be time for a change. Perhaps we need to revitalize ourselves.

By formulating a vision, we can take risks, use our creative talents, convince others, and keep pursuing our dreams. We can be energized, and we can make a difference. We may have ideas about how the staffing mix could be more effective, how nurses could better collaborate with other members of the healthcare team, or how technology can be used to better improve patient outcomes. Any of these ideas could be the groundwork for our vision or our dream. Sometimes an idea that starts out as one person's "pet peeve" or "personal agenda"—a computer in every home or school, helping the poorest of the poor, or achieving racial equality—can, if communicated effectively, become a group's quest. However one looks at it, one person's dream can excite others to follow or to envision their own separate piece of a larger vision. It seems that people who have dreams want to make a difference and are willing to do whatever it takes to fulfill those dreams. They believe that it is better to risk potential chaos or even failure than to accept the status quo. In other words, they are leaders in the fullest sense of the term.

Kouzes and Posner (1995, p. 120) suggest potential leaders use the following framework when developing a vision:

- Think first about your past.
- Determine what you want.
- Write an article about how you've made a difference.
- Write a short vision statement.
- Act on your intuition.
- Test your assumptions.
- Become a futurist.
- Rehearse with visualizations and affirmations.

For example, a graduate student in nursing decides to apply for a scholarship. The application asks for the usual information about previous work, grade point average, memberships in professional organizations, and so forth. It then requests that applicants share why they think they should be awarded a scholarship. Using Kouzes and Posner's (1995) framework, this student might focus her application on the following points, emphasizing how they make her an excellent candidate to receive this award. Her work as a staff nurse is described in terms of patient outcomes. She notes the creative teams on which she was a member or that she led. She describes research with which she assisted and the protocols she helped develop. She articulates clearly her reasons for pursuing the role and for which this particular graduate program will prepare her, specifically relating those goals to what she currently does in practice, what topics she will be studying, and what issues she will be researching. She integrates this information into a short vision statement of how this graduate program will prepare her for her ideal job. She mentions that she is submitting one of her papers as a manuscript for publication. She shares her insights about the healthcare system and explains how she thinks she can really make a difference, using examples to maximize her viewpoints. She concludes by writing her goals upon graduation and her expectations after 3 and 5 years. Such an application—with a clearly articulated vision—is likely to be reviewed quite positively by the scholarship selection committee as well as serve as a professional guide for this nurse to ascribe to during the next few years of working on her graduate degree.

What Happens If There Is No Vision?

When people wander aimlessly through their professional and personal lives, they tend not to accomplish the same results as those who are more focused. They may not take advantage of opportunities for professional growth because they were unaware of such opportunities, they did not think they could "measure up" and be successful, chose to fulfill a personal goal (e.g., a "vacation of a lifetime") instead, or did not wish to invest the time and energy needed to succeed.

Manfredi (1995) described what she called the art of legendary leadership by telling a story that depicts what can happen if one does not have a vision. Many years ago when the long-term mayor of a village passed away, the town elders gathered to select a successor. They asked for volunteers and after awhile, three candidates were found. There were no job description or selection criteria, so the elders decided to test the candidates' leadership by placing each in charge of the village for one month. The most successful candidate would become the mayor. One candidate believed he should keep the village stable and espoused the motto, "No need to grow, support the status quo." The town was so bored they let this candidate go. The second candidate believed one must create structure in order to lead, so he developed many rules and regulations to be followed by the people (but not by their leader). Not agreeing with this perspective, the elders had a bonfire and burned all 700 volumes of rules that this candidate had developed. The third candidate believed leaders know what is best for the people and the villagers cannot be trusted to make decisions or develop ideas, so he made all the decisions and never consulted anyone. After one month of such rule, the elders decided this candidate also was not suitable. But what to do? All three candidates were rejected. The elders could not come to an agreement as to exactly what the role of a leader should be, so they went off and discussed this for awhile. They finally came up with five roles for a leader to possess: "Leaders create visions, leaders create climates, leaders create conflict, leaders create change, and leaders create leaders" (p. 62). Basically, if a person or group does not have a vision, he or she cannot create a climate for conflict, change, and growth. Without conflict, change, and growth, new leaders will not be able to emerge from the group to inspire further conflict, change, and growth, and "the status quo will be perpetuated" by the leader who "knows best for the group" and creates many "rules and regulations."

Who Should Participate in Vision Development?

Bennis (1994) believed that one can learn how to develop a vision, and Manfredi (1995) made the point that anyone, not only the leader, can initiate an idea that is visionary. Everyone needs to integrate her/his individual goals to create an overall vision for a group or organization. For example, a unit with nurses who are attempting to create more evidence-based protocols, use research-based data, and improve care quality can form an Evidence-Based Practice Committee that meets monthly and an active online communication forum to facilitate participation by all staff in accomplishing the vision of providing evidence based practice.

It is the idea that sparks a vision that is the most significant part of developing a vision; and we all have had creative ideas that have been of great interest to others. Sometimes one individual will express a thought, someone else will add to it, and another person will expand it even more. Soon the entire group is involved in creating the idea. When this happens, change is likely to occur quickly or with minimal barriers. This process can occur when nurses want to develop a new approach to staffing, a philosophy of patient care, or a new nursing-driven protocol. For example, a group of staff nurses are discussing the challenges presented by maintaining the intravenous lines of patients with hard-to-stick veins. One nurse says how difficult she finds having to insert a new line every 4 hours, hurt the patient, and explain to the patient and family over and over again why a restick is necessary. Another nurse suggests that perhaps nurses should have a voice in determining which patients receive routine intravenous access and which receive a more invasive line. Someone else then asserts that nurses should insert the peripherally inserted central catheter (PICC) and manage the patients who have these more invasive lines. The entire group then goes on to talk about quality patient care in general. Thus the idea of providing nurses with more independence regarding intravenous fluid and medication administration served as the starting point for an even bigger dream— have significantly more nurse-driven protocols so that higher-quality, more cost-effective care could be delivered. In nursing, the direct care providers typically are most aware of what is best for the patient and what would improve the way care is delivered. Such nurses have ideas, dreams, and visions. Sadly, however, they often fail to do anything significant about them. Although it generally falls to the leader to actually implement a vision, everyone in the group needs to be involved to achieve success.

In a classic article on leaders and vision, Zaleznik (1989) suggested two ways to influence people: (1) help them realize that the proposed change will advance their interests, and (2) influence them to want to succeed for the group/organization, not just for self-recognition and promotion. Both the leader and the followers, therefore, need to be immersed in the process of formulating the vision and integrating it into the day-to-day work of the group. Throughout this process, the leader needs to be available to followers to help them clarify the vision, see how their efforts contribute to the vision, and be passionate about working toward the vision.

Strategies to Assist People with Vision Development

Having positive experience with trying new things, being involved in new opportunities, and being encouraged to take risks will assist with vision development. In 1991 Sarah Weddington, past counsel for *Roe v. Wade*, delivered a keynote address at the National League for Nursing Annual Convention in which she shared several ideas on how to gain practice in leading. The major focus of her presentation was that a leader must be passionate about what he or she does and must always strive to accomplish his or her dream. The dream must be a product of the ideal and what would have the most positive impact for the future. This perspective clarifies that to be effective, a vision must encompass many perspectives, it also must be future oriented. Leaders, therefore, must be proactive and not shy away from new things. Rather, they need to take time to try different ways, think about things in a new fashion, and have the confidence to encourage others to share the dream.

Koestenbaum (2002) offers an analysis of what he thinks it takes for people to be successful leaders and how to achieve specific goals. His book, in essence, is a compilation of how to create environments and societies that will facilitate the achievement of goals. Koestenbaum describes his Leadership Diamond Model, which revolves around the concepts of time, democracy, motivation, teamwork, and salesmanship. When analyzing one's leadership ability and/or contemplating developing new visions, using these concepts to visualize the plan is helpful.

Cohen (2004) emphasizes the importance of being aware of environmental influences and how it sometimes is necessary to change strategy or components of a strategy in order to fulfill goals. He also reminds us that the success of strategy depends on the "judgment and leadership qualities of the individual responsible for the undertaking" (p. vii). He offers 10 essential principles that are helpful when developing and carrying out one's vision:

- Commit fully to a goal.
- Seize the initiative and keep it.
- Economize to best use your resources.
- Use strategic positioning.
- Do the unexpected.
- Keep things simple.
- Prepare multiple, simultaneous alternatives.
- Take the indirect route to your objective.
- Practice timing and sequencing.
- Exploit your success.

Cohen describes realistic examples of strategizing both successfully and unsuccessfully and offers reasonable ideas of how to examine one's plan and make changes mid-stream and in crises so success is the most potential outcome.

> *Harry Truman was right, it's the leaders who shape history. There would have been no United States without Thomas Jefferson, no Third Reich without Adolph Hitler. But no man or woman becomes a leader unless he or she wants to. They've got to have a burning need to get there.* —Robert Ludlum (in The Icarus Agenda, p. 264)

One can learn how to communicate a vision in an articulate and persuasive manner. Conger (1989) suggests that the leader use metaphors and analogies to excite others and that the leader stimulate multiple senses (intellect, emotions, values, and imagination) simultaneously. Abraham Lincoln's powerful words in the Gettysburg Address—"government of the people, for the people, and by the people"—had a much greater impact than if he had said, "government of, for, and by the people" (Conger, 1989, p. 169). Franklin Delano Roosevelt tended to use folk imagery to share his ideas with the citizenry, and he used sports analogies in his fireside chats (Conger, 1989, p. 81); both were things with which people could easily relate. Another example of someone who related well at the grassroots level and established trust was Lee Iacocca, former CEO of Chrysler. Iacocca expressed his dream to rebuild the car company and his willingness to give everything it would take when he announced that he would accept a $1.00 salary for the whole year. Such a strategy created a strong identification between Iacocca and the average Chrysler employee, and it demonstrated an extraordinary level of personal commitment to a vision (Conger, 1989, pp. 73–74). In fact, more and more leaders are appreciating the importance of having commitment and passion for work and are "re-infusing passion, zest, and spirit into the workplace" (Bolman & Deal, 2001, p. 6), so that over time a bottom-line focus does not take a toll on employees' motivation, loyalty, and performance.

Although some leaders may be inclined to try to convince others with impressive numbers, Conger (1989) asserts that statistical summaries are uninformative and lack impact because they are colorless. He suggested brief face-to-face comments as being most substantial in getting people to buy into an idea, pursue a vision, or make a change. Other speech techniques such as repetition, rhythm, and alliteration are effective in helping articulate one's vision, as is evident in Martin Luther King, Jr.'s "I Have a Dream" speech. Conger also suggests that one use a loud volume, some body movements, and complete sentences with few pauses between them. It also is helpful to avoid "I think," "I guess," "please," and "thank you." Focusing on the basic message portrays the leader as confident, effective, and someone others would want to follow. In essence, leaders must be able to communicate their vision effectively, a skill that many believe is the most important characteristic of being a leader (Bennis & Nanus, 1985; Nanus, 1992).

Nurses today are knowledgeable and sophisticated. Therefore, nurse leaders must be able to communicate a clear vision but be open to the team's ideas regarding how the vision can be realized. A framework of skills is needed to be successful in articulating, communicating, and propelling a vision. Senge (2006) says a leader, particularly one in the healthcare arena, must be a systems thinker, have shared visioning, facilitate team learning, and have personal mastery. Champy (1995) agrees with Senge's list of competencies for healthcare leaders and adds skills of association, collaboration, communication, and mobilizing others. Drucker (1989) reaffirmed these descriptions of a leader when he articulated the skills of envisioning, coaching, knowing technology, and facilitating. All three of these organizational behaviorists agree on the necessity of a leader having and being able to clearly and effectively communicate the dream, the vision.

Look before you leap . . . or you'll find yourself behind. —Benjamin Franklin

An analogy serves to summarize these ideas about vision. A sailor is returning to port in the middle of a thunderstorm with barely 3 feet of visibility. The best thing the sailor can do is to concentrate on the ultimate destination, not on every foot of sea between him and land. This metaphor can be used in describing the journey a group, organization, or professional takes in reaching a dream. One must constantly look forward even if it takes a long time and a great deal of work and energy to get there. To "keep on track," the leader must help all members of the group feel a sense of ownership and be creative throughout the process of moving toward the vision.

THE PROCESS OF CREATIVITY

The essence of creativity is having the ability to play (Bennis, 1994). Creativity "demands intuition, uncertainty, unconventionality, and individual expression" (Conger, 1989, p. 17). Creativity, as it relates to leaders, occurs when leaders review their experiences to create new ideas (Valiga & Bruderle, 1997). Leadership is about "creating a new way of life" and changing the "business as usual environment" (Kouzes & Posner, 1993, pp. 37–39). If chaos describes our current reality, as many experts claim (discussed in Chapter 7), creativity is one skill we will need to appreciate, develop, and incorporate to successfully navigate this white-water turbulence. When unexpected events happen, leaders need to use them as learning experiences and not block learning by perceiving surprises as always negative happenings (McDaniel, Jordan, & Fleeman, 2003).

Creativity involves believing that "there is no one answer that is right but many answers that might work" (Wheatley & Kellner-Rogers, 1996, p. 16). As nurses we must re-frame how we think about our work so that we are more creative, open to a variety of possibilities, and open to options that might lead to successful outcomes. It is always conceivable that some of our options may not work the way we visualize them, but after observing new methods of providing care and determining they are not feasible, we will discover new options that, with some work and feedback from the team, will suggest even "better" options. These new ideas would never have been created if trying different options was not attempted.

Perhaps nurses need to become more involved in developing programs for outpatients to attend, writing grants to obtain funding for health promotion programs, educating larger groups of patients, trying different staff mix patterns, being more flexible with time schedules to include 9- or 7-hour shifts depending on unit needs, developing healthcare policies, serving on political action boards, and any number of other activities that will improve healthcare for people. In other words, nurses will have to become more comfortable with ambiguity and uncertainty so that they can see "new forms take shape, new ideas develop, and new goals fulfilled" (Valiga & Bruderle, 1997, p. 234). Most probably, it is easier to increase creativity by changing conditions in the work setting or home atmosphere than by influencing people to think in a more creative fashion (Csikszentmihalyl, 1996). In other words, it may be easier and more effective to focus on providing a creative ambiance in schools, day-care centers, homes, churches, and work settings than to focus on the process of thinking creatively.

More often than not, leaders are made, not born, and they accept that the growth process includes making mistakes (Bennis, 1994). This has relevance for the individual nurse who is a leader or an effective follower. It is no longer acceptable for nurses to deal only with the here and now of a specific patient assignment in the hospital or home setting. Nurse leaders need to partner with the patient and form alliances with family members, community groups, and other healthcare professionals to provide health teaching, promote self-competence for the patient, and gather relevant data to determine whether desired outcomes are being realized. It is time to change our belief that what we have known is all there is, and it is time to change our belief that how things are done has to be the way things continue to be done. Wheatley and Kellner-Rogers (1996, pp. 13–14) challenge us with the following beliefs about life creating itself:

Everything is in a constant process of discovery and creating. Everything is changing all of the time: individuals, systems, environments, the rules, and the processes of evolution. Even change changes. Every organism reinterprets the rules, creates exceptions for itself, and creates new rules.

Life uses messes to get to well-ordered solutions. Life doesn't seem to share our desires for efficiency or neatness. It uses redundancy, fuzziness, dense webs of relationships, and unending trials and errors to find what works.

Life is intent on finding what works, not what's right. It is the ability to keep finding solutions that are important; any one solution is temporary. There are no permanently right answers. The capacity to keep changing, to find what works now, is what keeps any organism alive.

Life creates more possibilities as it engages with opportunities. There are no "windows of opportunity," narrow openings in the fabric of space-time that soon disappear forever. Possibilities beget more possibilities; they are infinite.

Life is attracted to order. It experiments until it discovers how to form a system that can support diverse members. Individuals search out a wide range of possible relationships to discover whether they can organize into a life-sustaining system. These explorations continue until a system is discovered. This system then provides stability for its members, so that individuals are less buffered by change.

Life organizes around identity. Every living thing acts to develop and preserve itself. Identity is the filter that every organism or system uses to make sense of the world. New information, new relationships, changing environments—all are interpreted through a sense of self. This tendency toward self-creation is so strong that it creates a seeming paradox. An organism will change to maintain its identity.

Everything participates in the creation and evolution of its neighbors. There are no unaffected outsiders. No one system dictates conditions to another. All participate together in creating the conditions of their interdependence.

Obviously, there is no one right answer to most situations. There is no way anyone can plan for all of the potential problems that might occur when attempting to institute creative and innovative approaches to reach a vision, and there is no room for an "everything has to be right" attitude. It makes no sense waiting for everything to be "just right" before we act because things will continue to change and some sort of acceptable order will emerge.

Perhaps as nurses we should develop our right brain skills more so that we can be more intuitive, conceptual, and artistic instead of being dominated by the left side of the brain with our logical planning, to-do lists, and conservative perspective. Bennis (1994) suggested we be whole-brained so that both concrete and abstract ideas can be used. For example, the mindmap of creativity (Fig. 5–2) depicts various actions that a creative person uses. Mindmapping is a method of note taking that could be effective in stimulating our creativity and developing our right-brain skills, as well as stimulating the flow of ideas from our more concrete left brain. This exercise of illustrating what one reads or sees may be a helpful exercise in developing the whole brain.

Think back to when you were in first grade. How do you think your teacher would have reacted if you gave an answer such as the one shown in Figure 5–3? For most of us, the teacher probably would have scolded us for being too right-brained! Nurse educators can assist the profession by designing learning experiences that allow for student creativity and the use of skills governed by both the right and left sides of the brain. In this way, nursing will achieve a better balance of task-oriented left-brain thinkers and creative right-brain thinkers.

Nurses also must focus less energy on and worry less about some unknown future; instead, we should focus more on the opportunities before us today and the possibilities awaiting us tomorrow. Thinking more openly, being more aware of possibilities, and being less structured and more creative will take us a long way. "If we believe that the world is self-organizing, then we don't have to be the organizers; in fact, we don't have to struggle to create networks, affiliations, or teams, . . . groups will just happen" (Wheatley & Kellner-Rogers, 1996, p. 35). The following case study illustrates this point.

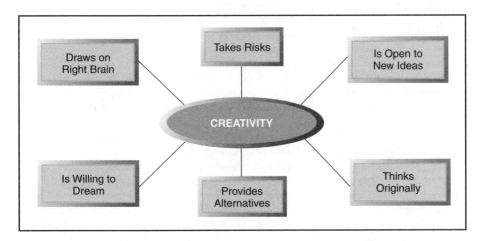

FIGURE 5-2 · Mindmap of creativity.

FIGURE 5-3 • Using our right brain.

Case Study: Development of a Vision Using Creativity

The following case depicts how nurses were able to use their creative abilities and energize themselves and colleagues by following their dream.

There was much unhappiness and low morale on the trauma unit where a group of nurses were employed. It was related to strictly enforced role limitations for RNs. Due to the multiple residents rotating through their unit, it was difficult to gain new skills, communicate with physicians, and collaborate with the Intensivists about the challenging cases. The nurse manager was not interested in having an Acute Care Nurse Practitioner, and constantly blocked any ideas to hire one. The unit was fairly noncollaborative with the physicians. Nurses took orders from the doctors and were not encouraged to discuss their perceptions or share their knowledge about individual patients.

Three nurses on the unit were interested in becoming Acute Care Nurse Practitioners so they could achieve more autonomy in their practice. They were matriculated in the same master's program and just starting their clinical component. The hospital's policy was that staff should not do their student rotations at their place of employment, if possible. So, each student was at the other Level 1 trauma hospital in the city. These three nurse practitioner students observed the role of the RN at this other institution had a larger practice scope than their role as an RN. Because the RN's role was expanded, their student Nurse Practitioner role was also expanded and created opportunities for growth that they had never expected. The three students developed and communicated a new vision for their unit with their colleagues, which allowed for an upgrading of the RN role and empowered the RN staff to dispel the "handmaiden mentality."

The staff, led by the three nurse practitioner students, generated multiple changes and soon had an impact on the culture of the unit to such a degree that the nurse manager transferred to another position out of the critical care area. One of the students applied and was promoted to the nurse manager position and led the nurses in creating goals, accomplishing them, gaining new skills and responsibilities, creating new Acute Care Nurse Practitioner roles, and restructuring the unit to become a collaborative practice model. This unit's progress was a result of a team effort, which created a new vision and empowered staff to step up to a new role that eventually involved the entire unit. This is an example of how three nurses' efforts encouraged a whole unit to have ownership in the change process by being energetic, excited, and enthusiastic.

So in healthcare today, the mergers, acquisitions, affiliations, and partnering are really not a bad thing but a natural force; a bringing together of talent, resources and, one hopes, better patient outcomes. Our ability to be creative and use networking will ultimately allow us to survive. We must foster rethinking, discovery, and curiosity as they support change. This is the new way of thinking about leadership, and we have to change our way of thinking about our responsibilities. "In a self-organizing system, people do for themselves most of what in the past has been done to them. Self-organizing systems create their own structures, patterns of behavior, and processes for accomplishing their work. They design what is necessary to do the work. They agree on behaviors and relationships that make sense to them. Those of us not directly involved in the doing of their work can give up fussing about designs, believing that our timelines make things happen, or that our training programs change the behavior of the organization" (Wheatley & Kellner-Rogers, 1996, p. 38). We can support and trust one another, and create possibilities or dreams never thought of before, if we can give up the need to organize every tiny detail, allow ourselves to be creative, use our ingenuity, and collaborate with others to maximize our creativity.

The Significance of Creativity

Creativity is necessary if nurses are to effectively manage the multitude of changes occurring in healthcare today and that are expected to continue well into the future. "Partnering" is a buzzword that to most nurses means a change in responsibilities or a loss of job. Perhaps if more nurses were entrepreneurs, our profession could undergo some serious growth despite the current environment. Porter-O'Grady (1997) describes how he has succeeded in the role of a consultant and entrepreneur. He shares that the secret of his career has been good mentors, seizing the opportunity to try something new even when he was not sure he was prepared for it, and accepting changes in his professional and personal life. His recommendation to fellow nurses is to gather practice and skills in leadership and design new ways of managing patient care delivery. Being willing to try new things, challenge traditional ways of thinking and behaving, and being open to new ways of thinking will broaden our visions. We cannot let ourselves accept that all "flowers are red [and] green leaves are green" (Chapin, 1978). The words to Harry Chapin's song "Flowers Are Red," illustrate what can happen when individuals are not allowed to think creatively. Creativity allows us to accomplish our visions with excitement and enthusiasm. One gets a resurgence of energy when something new and exciting occurs, or when one has an "a-ha" insight. This energy also comes from change itself, and when that change relates to our work and what we do, we can experience phenomenal growth. "Work comes from the inside out, work is an expression of our soul, our inner being. It's unique to the individual, it's creative" (Fox, 1994, p. 49). Work, therefore, should not be boring, repetitious, tiring, and frustrating. Instead, it should be and can be energizing, challenging, rewarding, and growth producing.

Using Creativity

Nurses have the capacity to use their creative talents to staff units in new ways, research new protocols, administer medications and treatments differently, communicate patient information to other professionals more powerfully, develop materials to market nurses' skills for patients at home, implement support groups for inpatients and outpatients, or build partnerships with clinics or school-based healthcare providers. For too long, nurses have been accustomed to staying in the same environment (home, long-term care facility, school, clinic, or hospital) for their entire career. As new roles emerge and new settings provide opportunities for nurses, there is no need to feel stuck or to be stuck. Nurses are becoming more independent as they practice autonomously and in multiple environments. Today, nurses are vital members of multidisciplinary health team efforts, willing to do things differently, revising protocols to be more patient-oriented, focusing more on measuring patient outcomes, and acting on their concerns about providing quality, cost-effective care.

Zander and Zander (2000) suggest that the way each person sees the world is a reflection of whether we see through glasses of scarcity or possibility. If more nurses could use the half-full glass perspective rather than the half-empty glass one, they could serve as powerful role models for future nurses. One study (Grossman, 2004a), in fact, demonstrated this very clearly. In a shadowing experience where students ($N = 182$) were assigned to work alongside mentor nurses, the researcher found that if the mentor was positive in her thinking, creative in finding new ways to do things, and visionary/goal-oriented, students reported having a productive and growth-producing clinical experience.

In another study (Grossman, 2004b), students analyzed their own creativity scores using the "How Creative Are You?" tool (Raudsepp, 1981) prior to and after the leadership rotation. (Note: This instrument is included in the Critical Thinking Exercises at the end of this chapter.) The findings include the following: (1) 87% of all students in this study ($N = 72$) had low creativity scores pre-rotation; (2) 45% of the students perceived their mentors as consistently displaying positive thinking, being creative, and being visionary; (3) 38% of students with the positive role models experienced statistically significant higher creativity scores post-rotation; and (4) students not assigned to a positive role model had very little change in their creativity score post-rotation. Thus, having a creative and positive thinking mentor did influence the students' perception of how they viewed their creativity, and perhaps this experience will enhance their ability to be creative.

McCall (1989) suggested some interesting methods by which leaders can use creative strategies to clarify and achieve their visions. By being "feisty," leaders can deliberately create conflicts to spark new ideas between selected, key people and propel their ideas forward. Creative leaders also are "crafty" in that they are politically astute, know how to increase their power base, and can enlist broad support for creative, different pursuits. If creative leaders are to survive, they must be able to disassociate with failure and associate with success. Being creative puts a leader in a bit of danger because it involves taking risks. Using standards of excellence also characterizes a creative leader because one would have to be very demanding to help everyone involved with the new idea meet the highest, most impeccable standards. McCall (1989) also asserted that a creative leader has to act before thinking, rather than think before acting, and has to be inconsistent so that the leader can keep the system "open" for new ideas and changes. Last, creative leaders must use intuition and hunches so that they do not miss a potentially new way to accomplish the vision. By using these strategies in any nursing role, it would be difficult to become bored with a job, to burn out, or to feel stuck.

CONCLUSION

There is no doubt that leaders must be passionate about their visions, their dreams of making a significant difference or bettering the world. It is also crucial that leaders be able to persuade people to "grab on" to this vision and become involved in creating change. As Zaleznik (1989) noted, "one cannot be successful without using one's imagination and without being more comfortable with disorder and chaos. In other words, we need to avoid the 'If it ain't broke, don't fix it' way of thinking" (p. 62). Change will occur no matter what we do to maintain the existing order. If we have articulated worthy visions, if we have allowed ourselves to become comfortable with the notion of creativity, and if we use creative strategies to achieve our vision, we will thrive from this change, grow personally, and be effective leaders who shape a better world.

Vision is the art of seeing things invisible. —Jonathan Swift

CRITICAL THINKING EXERCISES

Read the story "Footprints." How does this relate to creativity? To leadership? To providing leadership and fostering creativity in nursing?

Footprints

In a faraway land long ago, there was once a wise and good village chief who had a most exciting announcement. "Of utmost importance," he reminded his villagers, "is the ability to travel to the port to trade our jewelry for food. Until recently those traveling to the port simply left our village and wandered aimlessly until they either found the port or died. I am happy to announce that thanks to the efforts of our wise and most scientific medicine man we have captured the essence of travel. We have discovered that all travel is based on footprints. Follow footprints precisely and you will never get lost going to or from the port again."

"But what about trees?" asked one villager.

"Trees are not footprints, and trees should be ignored," replied the chief.

"May we consider the stars?" questioned another.

"Don't be foolish," commanded the chief. "What could be farther from footprints than stars? Have I not told you already? There is no travel without footprints. Footprints are the essence of travel. Understand footprints, and the concept of travel is yours forever. You will never be lost again."

That was many years ago. And since that time many villagers have come and gone from the port, never taking their eyes off the footprints. Some of the more scholarly villagers over the years have studied and refined footprintology, writing long, scholarly discourses on the many things that footprints show, and of the many truths to be found through scrutiny of footprints.

Over the years the methods of observing footprints have been refined to such an exact science that many years of studying with rigorous examinations are required to truly practice and teach footprintology. In fact, before each young man is able to leave the village he must be thoroughly educated in footprintology as the essence of travel, lest some day he look up at the trees or stars and lose sight of that essence that the wisest of wise know as travel.

Source: Bagley, D. (1979). Footprints (a parable about knowledge). *Journal of Creative Behavior, 13* (4), 286–287.

_____

_____

What is your vision for nursing in general? In your current sphere of practice? What goals do you have for the profession? Which of these goals can be achieved by nurses themselves, and which need external support or action?

_____

_____

Envision your professional goals for the near future and for 3 years down the road from now. Imagine your long-term goals. Given the chaotic healthcare system and changes the nursing profession is experiencing, think about how you need to design your career in order to realize these long-term visions.

_____

_____

Think about your current leadership ability. How can you maximize these skills so you will be able to accomplish your professional goals and increase your impact on the healthcare system?

_____

_____

Using Martin Luther King, Jr.'s "I Have a Dream" speech (See Web site *http://www.mecca. org/~crights/dream.html*) or the speeches of other powerful orators (e.g., John F. Kennedy, Margaret Thatcher, Abraham Lincoln), identify communication methods you could use to articulate your dream clearly.

_____

_____

Compare and contrast an experience you've had professionally to Harry Chapin's song "Flowers Are Red." How could you use "every color" to prevent a recurrence? (See Web site *http://www.songlyrics4u.com/harry-chapin/flowers-are-red.html*)

_____

_____

Create a mind map of leadership.

_____

_____

Sternberg's (2007) Systems Model of Leadership incorporates wisdom, creativity, and intelligence. Using this model, describe how you generate a new idea, evaluate if the idea is good, implement the idea to maximize performance, and use your knowledge and experience to evaluate its effectiveness.

_____

_____

Complete the "How Creative Are You?" questionnaire. What did you learn about yourself?

_____

_____

HOW CREATIVE ARE YOU?

Directions. Following are 30 statements that are useful in determining a person's current level of creativity. Read each statement. Answer "**A**" for those statements with which you "Agree." Answer "**B**" for those statements on which you are "In Between" or "Don't Know." Answer "**C**" for those with which you "Disagree."

1. I always work with a great deal of certainty that I'm following the correct procedures for solving a particular problem. _____

2. It would be a waste of time for me to ask questions if I had no hope of obtaining answers. _____

3. I concentrate harder on what interests me than do most people. _____

4. I feel that a logical step-by-step method is best for solving problems. _____

5. I occasionally voice opinions in groups that seem to turn people off.

6. It is more important for me to do what I believe to be right than to try to win the approval of others. _____

7. I need to have things interesting and exciting. _____

8. I am able to stick with difficult problems over extended periods of time. _____

9. On occasion I get overly enthusiastic about things. _____

10. I often get my best ideas when doing nothing in particular. _____

11. I rely on intuitive hunches and the feeling of "rightness" or "wrongness" when moving toward the solution of a problem. _____

12. I like hobbies that involve collecting things. _____

13. Daydreaming has provided the impetus for many of my more important projects. _____

14. I have a high degree of aesthetic sensitivity. _____

15. I am driven to achieve positions or situations of power in life. _____

16. I like people who are most sure of their conclusions. _____

17. Inspiration has nothing to do with successful solution of problems. _____

18. I am much more interested in coming up with new ideas than I am trying to sell them to others. _____

19. I would enjoy spending an entire day alone, just "chewing the mental cud." _____

20. I tend to avoid situations in which I might feel inferior. _____

21. I resent things being uncertain and unpredictable. _____

22. I like people who follow the rule, "business before pleasure." _____

23. Self-respect is much more important than the respect of others. _____

24. I feel that people who strive for perfection are unwise. _____

25. I prefer to work with others in a team effort rather than solo. _____

26. I like work in which I must influence others. _____

27. Many problems that I encounter in life cannot be resolved in terms of right or wrong solutions. _____

28. It is important for me to have a place for everything, everything in its place. _____

29. I prefer writers who write so that the average person can understand them to those who use strange or fancy words. _____

30. I would be more comfortable in a job that had a steady routine than I would in a job in which a person would have to do different things every day. _____

After having selected an "A," "B," or "C" response to each statement, follow the scoring instructions to determine your current level of creativity. To compute your score, circle your response to each statement and add up the value assigned to each item.

STATEMENT NUMBER	A	B	C
1.	0	1	2
2.	0	1	2
3.	4	1	2
4.	2	0	3
5.	2	1	0
6.	3	0	1
7.	3	0	1
8.	4	1	0
9.	3	0	1
10.	2	1	0
11.	4	0	2
12.	0	1	2
13.	3	0	1
14.	3	0	1
15.	0	1	2
16.	1	0	2
17.	0	1	3
18.	2	1	0
19.	2	0	1
20.	0	1	2
21.	0	1	2
22.	0	1	2
23.	3	0	-1
24.	1	0	2
25.	0	1	2

26.	1	2	2
27.	2	1	0
28.	0	1	2
29.	1	0	2
30.	1	1	3

Source: Raudsepp, E. (1981). *How creative are you?* New York: Putnam.

65–75 Exceptionally creative

49–64 Very creative

30–48 Above average

16–29 Average

8–15 Below average

15–7 Uncreative

References

Bagley, D. (1979). Footprints (A parable about knowledge). *Journal of Creative Behavior, 13*(4), 286–287.

Bennis, W. (1994). *On becoming a leader* (2nd ed.). Reading, MA: Addison-Wesley.

Bennis, W., & Nanus, B. (1985). *Leaders: The strategies for taking charge.* New York: Harper & Row.

Bolman, L., & Deal, T. (2001). *Leading with soul: An uncommon journey of spirit* (2nd ed). San Francisco: Jossey-Bass.

Champy, J. (1995). *Reengineering management.* New York: Harper Business.

Chapin, H. (1978). Flowers are red. *Legends of the lost and found album.* New York: Electra/Asylum Records, Division of Warner Communications. Accessed August, 2 ,2007 from, *http://www.songlyrics4u.com/harry-chapin/flowers-are-red.html*

Cohen, W. (2004). *The art of the strategist: 10 essential principles for leading your company to victory.* New York: American Management Associates.

Conger, J. (1989). *The charismatic leader: Behind the mystique of exceptional leadership.* San Francisco: Jossey-Bass.

Covey, S. (2004). *The 8th habit: From effectiveness to greatness.* New York: Free Press.

Csikszentmihalyl, M. (1996). *Creativity flow and the psychology of discovery and intervention.* New York: HarperCollins.

Drucker, P. (1989). *The new realities: In government and politics/in economics and business/in society and world view.* New York: Harper & Row.

Fox, M. (1994). *Reinvention of work: A new vision of livelihood for our time.* San Francisco: Harper.

Grossman, S. (2004a). Developing leadership through shadowing a leader in health care. In H. Feldman & M. Greenberg (Eds.), *Educating for leadership.* New York: Springer.

Grossman, S. (2004b). Variables impacting leadership development. Unpublished manuscript. School of Nursing, Fairfield University, Fairfield, CT.

King, M. (1963). I have a dream. Accessed August 2, 2007 from, *http://www.mecca.org/ ~crights/dream.html*

Koestenbaum, P. (2002). *Leadership The inner side of greatness*. San Francisco: Jossey-Bass.

Kotter, J. (1990). *A force for change*. New York: The Free Press.

Kouzes, J., & Posner, B. (1993). *Credibility: How leaders gain and lose it, why people demand it*. San Francisco: Jossey-Bass.

Kouzes, J., & Posner, B. (1995). *The leadership challenge*. San Francisco: Jossey-Bass.

LeJoly, E. (1983). *Mother Teresa of Calcutta*. New York: Harper & Row.

Manes, S., & Andrews, P. (1993). *Gates: How Microsoft's mogul reinvented an industry and made himself the richest man in America*. New York: Doubleday.

Manfredi, C. (1995). The art of legendary leadership: Lessons for new and aspiring leaders. *Nursing Leadership Forum, 1*(2), 62–64.

McCall, M. (1989). Conjecturing about creative leaders. In W. E. Rosenbach & R. L. Taylor (Eds.), *Contemporary issues in leadership* (2nd ed.) (pp. 111–120). Boulder, CO: Westview Press.

McDaniel, R., Jordan, M., & Fleeman, B. (2003). Surprise, surprise, surprise! A complexity science view of the unexpected. *Health Care Management Review, 28*(3), 266–278.

Mintzberg, H. (2004). *Managers, not MBAs*. San Francisco: Berrett-Koehler.

Nanus, B. (1992). *Visionary leadership*. San Francisco: Jossey-Bass.

Parse, R. (1997). Leadership: The essentials. (Editorial). *Nursing Science Quarterly, 10*(3), 109.

Porter-O'Grady, T. (1997). The private practice of nursing: The gift of entrepreneurialism. *Nursing Administration Quarterly, 22*(1), 23–29.

Porter-O'Grady, T., & Wilson, C. (1995). *The leadership revolution in health care: Altering systems, changing behaviors*. Gaithersburg, MD: Aspen.

Raudsepp, E. (1981). *How creative are you?* New York: Putnam.

Sashkin, M. (1989). Visionary leadership: A perspective from education. In W. E. Rosenbach & R. L. Taylor (Eds.), *Contemporary issues in leadership* (2nd ed.) (pp. 222–234). Boulder, CO: Westview Press.

Senge, P. (2006). *The fifth discipline: The art and practice of the learning organization* (2nd ed.). New York: Doubleday Currency.

Sternberg, H. (2007). A systems model of leadership. *American Psychologist, 62*(1), 34–42.

Stoltz, P. (2000). *Adversity quotient at work*. New York: Morrow.

Valiga, T., & Bruderle, E. (1997). *Using the arts and humanities to teach nursing: A creative approach*. New York: Springer.

Weddington, S. (1991). Leaders are made not born (The Novello Lecture). Presented at the National League for Nursing Convention, Nashville, TN, June 1991.

Wheatley, M., & Kellner-Rogers, M. (1996). *A simpler way*. San Francisco: Berrett-Koehler.

Zaleznik, A. (1989). Why managers lack vision. *Business Month, 8,* 59–64.

Zander, R., & Zander, B. (2000). *The art of possibility*. Boston: Harvard Business School Press.

CHAPTER 6

Gender Perspectives in Leadership

LEARNING OBJECTIVES
- Compare "feminine leadership" with "masculine leadership."
- Examine the concept of androgyny.
- Describe barriers women face to exercising leadership in organizations.
- Propose strategies that women and men can use to enhance their effectiveness as leaders in organizations.
- Compare "web" organizations with "hierarchical" ones.

INTRODUCTION

As has been noted, most of the studies about leaders and leadership have focused on men and the male perspective. Although this information is valuable and much of what we know about leadership—the need to have a vision, the reciprocal relationship between leaders and followers, the willingness to take risks, and so on—has broad applicability, it still is rooted largely in a "masculine" framework. There is a growing body of literature, however, that notes differences in the ways women lead (Austin, 2002; Babcock & Laschever, 2003; Felder, 1996; Gordon, 1991; Grunwald, 1992; Helgesen, 1990a; Klenke, 1996; Kram & Hampton, 1998; Lipman-Blumen, 1992; Long, 1998; May, 2001; Melia & Lyttle, 1986; Rosener, 1990; Schein, 1989). Because most nurses are women, understanding gender perspectives in leadership is an essential area of exploration.

This chapter explores some of the "typical stereotypes" about differences between men and women and how they translate into (1) differences in each gender's approach to leadership and (2) different types of organizational structures that best "fit" with

99

each approach. This chapter also examines ways in which the best of both worlds can be combined into a truly effective leader.

COMMON GENDER DIFFERENCES

Leaders reflect the values, norms, strengths, and weaknesses of their groups and, indeed, of the larger society. Although this is usually considered a strength and an advantage, it can present a challenge for a female leader functioning in "a man's world," and who may be sent to "Bully Broad Boot Camp" if she is too aggressive (Austin, 2002).

"Maleness" often is associated with concepts such as dominance, independence, objectivity, rationality, competitiveness, aggressiveness, boldness, decisiveness, toughness, being logical, and being "thing-oriented." Since these terms are often associated with leadership, masculine traits often are equated with effective leadership skills (Kellerman & Rhode, 2006; Stivers, 1991). "Femaleness," on the other hand, typically is associated with ideas that are not aligned with leadership, ideas such as compliance, dependence, emotionality, weakness, being accepting, passivity, nurturance, and being "people-oriented." Comparisons such as those noted in Table 6–1 often are made in jest, but the basis of them is all too real for women in many arenas.

TABLE 6-1 A Businessman Versus a Businesswoman

BUSINESSMAN	BUSINESSWOMAN
A businessman is aggressive.	A businesswoman is pushy.
A well-dressed businessman is fashionable.	A well-dressed businesswomen is a "clotheshorse."
He loses his temper because he's so involved with his job.	She's "bitchy."
He's a man of the world.	She's "been around."
He's confident.	She's conceited.
He drinks because of excessive work pressures.	She's a lush.
He's enthusiastic.	She's emotional.
He's careful about details.	She's picky.
He's depressed (or hung over), so everyone tiptoes past his office.	She's moody, so it must be "her time of the month."
He follows through.	She doesn't know when to quit.
He's firm.	She's stubborn.
He makes wise judgments.	She reveals her prejudices.
He isn't afraid to say what he thinks.	She's opinionated.
He exercises authority.	She's tyrannical.
He's discreet.	She's secretive.
He's a stern taskmaster.	She's difficult to work for.

Although it is no longer remarkable to find women in positions of authority, power, and leadership, most women in the workforce still are clustered at the bottom of the employment "heap" (e.g., clerical jobs and low-paying professional jobs). It also has been shown that most individuals with political influence are men, and organizational heads tend not to be women. One report (Brooks, 1983) noted that "rather than being trained for the new technologies, many [women] wind up being taught only to master a few specific data-processing tasks that cannot be easily trans-ferred" (p. 31). They are, therefore, limited in what they can do, the opportunities they can pursue, and the breadth or possibly even the significance of contributions they can make to an organization. Ultimately their opportunities for advancement, personal growth, and leadership are limited. "As of 1996, women filled nearly a third of all management roles, but the majority [were] positions with relatively little power and authority" (Klenke, 1996, p. 17). And in healthcare, "as of 1999, women simply [were] not present in senior management positions to the extent that we would expect when 85 percent of U.S. healthcare workers are female" (Robinson-Walker, 1999, p. 3). Some argue that this "gender divide" (Babcock & Laschever, 2003) is widening, but others claim women are making significant strides in providing leadership in our society.

Reasons why there have been a limited number of women exercising leadership are many. Society does not expect and value leadership in women, and they typically are not socialized as leaders. There are few women leader role models, and women who do try to exert strong leadership behaviors sometimes are discriminated against and not supported in those efforts. It also has been claimed that women fear success and that they are fearful of competition. While women typically are quite expert at multi-tasking and managing successfully with limited resources, they often are afraid to ask for things they need (Babcock & Laschever, 2003) and often are willing to settle for what they are given. In addition, it is common to see references to the "Queen Bee syndrome," in which women "at the top" want to be only with men, want to keep other women down, and downplay the concerns expressed by women who are trying to succeed with comments such as, "I did it without much help; why can't you?"

Many women, however, have challenged the "system," overcome fears, fought vigorously for resources, dealt with the "Queen Bees," and obtained the education, training, and skills needed to compete effectively and move into positions of power and leadership. As a result, these hard-working, ambitious women may be seen as a threat to men and to other women, and have their "every move scrutinized, dissected, poured over, interpreted and reinterpreted" (Austin, 2002, p. 57). Therefore, they need to invest energy into dealing with all the stereotype issues (e.g., being perceived as threats or as not being "real" women), as well as dealing with the issues inherent in the job itself (e.g., improving the bottom line or producing a product before the com-petition does).

The challenges that women face in pursuing leadership roles are clearly related to early socialization. Assumptions are made about what is appropriate for girls and boys (e.g., "boys don't cry or play with dolls," and "girls are emotional and prefer more isolated play activities rather than competitive team sports"). Relationships develop based on these assumptions; they become deeply ingrained over time through experiences such as school (American Association of University Women, 1992), and socialization along these lines continues throughout adulthood. It is the woman, for example, who is more likely to struggle to balance work, family responsibilities, and other commitments because—even though changes continue to be made toward greater sharing of responsibilities—our society continues to allow the male partner to emphasize the work or professional role while expecting the female partner to "do it all."

> *Women tend to stick it out too long and just try to work harder for recognition.* —Marie Wunsch

Women who attempt to break away from these stereotypes are often regarded as "deviant" (Vance, 1979). Deviance is thought to occur when an individual varies too widely from the norm and fails to obey group rules. It is considered essentially pathological and a symptom of social disorganization. Thus women who assert themselves as leaders may be viewed negatively by the larger society.

Even women who **do** achieve high positions may be viewed with less credibility and respect than their male counterparts, and male and female peers alike may criticize them. Women leaders also may be considered inferior and "second class." Despite these challenges, however, women bring a unique dimension to leadership roles.

WOMEN'S WAYS OF LEADING

Although distinctions between men and women often are outlined in a humorous way (as noted in Table 6–1), differences between their styles and the way they lead have been reported. For example, the "alpha" and "beta" types of leadership described by Levenstein (1981) may be aligned with masculine and feminine leadership. According to this author, alpha leadership is analytic, relies heavily on rationale, is quantitative, relies on hierarchical relationships, and favors engineered solutions. It is a style that thrives on competitive challenges and sees power as a goal. In comparison, beta leadership is intuitive, qualitative, and concerned about growth. It relies on support relationships and is future-oriented. It is a style in which power is seen as a means to a goal that has relevance for the members of the group and those served by the group, rather than a goal in and of itself or a means to a goal that has relevance only for the leader. Alpha leadership might be more closely aligned with a male perspective, and beta leadership might be more reflective of female leadership.

> *Transformational leadership feels right to women because it's not asking anything that they haven't done.* —Jacquelyn M. Belcher

Robinson-Walker's (1999) study of nearly 100 women and men responsible for managing a significant portion of America's healthcare supported such findings. In addition, she reported on work done by the sociologist Neuhauser who noted in 1988 that "'tribal' membership profoundly affects values and behavior within organizations, and the most basic tribes are those of males and females. Even if men and women share the same values, Neuhauser suggests their thinking is organized differently, which results in different expressions of that thinking" (Robinson-Walker, 1999, p. 29).

> *Women and leadership have always made for an uneasy alliance. —Nancy Austin*

Such differences in thinking and leadership styles can have significant ramifications, as was pointed out in a brief piece related to military force (*Sexes differ on military force*, 1985). This piece noted that having more women in the House and Senate could significantly alter decision-making in the American political arena. It reported on the work of two Canadian researchers who concluded that women were less likely than men to support funding for nuclear weapons and missile testing and more likely to favor deterrence through disarmament rather than a cold war. Men, these researchers noted, tended to be not only more "pro-force" than women but also tended to see military defense issues in more "simplistic terms." Women tended to view the same issues from a more complex, "holistic" perspective that included the "human dimension." The researchers concluded that men and women organized their thoughts differently: "If nothing else, males had a much simpler perspective on things and tended to see issues in black and white terms . . . but women saw shades of gray" (*Sexes differ on military force*, 1985, p. 7). Although cold war issues are not the major concern in our society that they were in 1985 when this report was issued, conflict, crisis, change, and war remain significant factors in our lives. Therefore the findings of this study regarding women's perspectives, their tendency to be more nurturing and "other-oriented," the factors that enter into their decision making, and the ways in which their thinking and potential leadership differ from men are worth noting.

Rosener (1990) described four major areas of difference in style exhibited by the women leaders she studied: (1) they tended to encourage participation; (2) they shared power and information quite readily; (3) they were concerned about enhancing the self-worth of others; and (4) they worked to energize others. This is consistent with other descriptions of women leaders as nurturing, caring, and intimate; it also is consistent in its contrast to descriptions of male leaders as valuing autonomy, objectivity, and fairness. Rosener's work also supports men's tendency to use the power of their position in transactional exchanges (e.g., exchanging rewards for services rendered or punishment for poor performance).

These differences are supported by Helgesen (1990a), whose research revealed several dimensions in which women offer perspectives and reflect values that are a source of their uniqueness and their strength. Women, she says, value "an attention to process instead of a focus on the bottom line; a willingness to look at how an action will affect other people instead of simply asking, 'What's in it for me?'; a concern for the wider needs of the community; a disposition to draw on personal, private sphere experience when dealing in the public realm; an appreciation of diversity; [and] an outsider's impatience with rituals and symbols of status that divide people who work together and so reinforce hierarchies" (pp. xx–xxi).

Such attributes of women leaders also were supported in a study of several hundred women in the Houston area (May, 2001). These researchers found that the following six factors emerged as the most important skills and attributes of leaders, as identified by the women who participated in the study:

- Personal integrity: being guided by ethical standards and a moral compass; being trustworthy and credible
- Strategic vision/action orientation: finding the path; seeing possibilities and the big picture; crafting and communicating a vision, a preferred future
- Team building/communication skills: building coalitions, teams, and consensus; communicating clearly and directly; promoting debate and encouraging discussion; acknowledging the contributions of everyone
- Management and technical competencies: making decisions; thinking critically; solving problems; being technically proficient
- People skills: demonstrating respect, cultural sensitivity, and an ability to inspire others; allowing followers to make mistakes; sharing information; advocating for others
- Personal survival skills: being politically sensitive; possessing an entrepreneurial spirit, being comfortable with competitiveness, self-direction, and self-reliance; demonstrating candor and courage

This study concluded that women need to view themselves as leaders with something to offer the community, for "when women 'sit at the table,' the manner of discussion changes and different priorities are frequently set [which] enable the discussion to become more inclusive" (p. 122).

In the continuation of his seminal work on megatrends, Naisbitt (1982) partnered with a female forecaster to address 10 "new directions" for the 1990s (Naisbitt & Aburdene, 1990). One of the trends they predicted for the last decade of the 20th century was that it would be the "decade of women in leadership" (p. 216). These authors asserted that as individuals and organizations continue to evolve, they demand true leadership—leadership that respects people, encourages individuals to grow and contribute significantly, inspires commitment, and "empower[s] people by sharing authority" (p. 219). The individual who will provide this kind of leadership is a "self-developer" (a term initially proposed by Maccoby, 1981), "an individual who values independence, dislikes bureaucracies, and seeks to balance work with other priorities like family and recreation" (Naisbitt & Aburdene, 1990, p. 221), as well as a "teacher, facilitator, and coach" (p. 227). Women, these authors say, are extremely well positioned to function in such roles.

> *A true leader has the confidence to stand alone, the courage to make tough decisions, and the compassion to listen to the needs of others. He does not set out to be a leader, but becomes one by the quality of his actions and the integrity of his intent. In the end, leaders are much like eagles ... they don't flock, you find them one at a time.* —Anonymous

Book (2000) agreed. In her study of 14 of the most powerful women in American business, she found that these organizational leaders fostered a more collegial environment, played down their own egos, led "from the ground up" (p. 235), and displayed empathy, all of which engendered loyalty from and the respect of those with whom they worked. This researcher concluded that while women were better at communicating, empowering others, and being positive, they also were "more decisive [and] better at planning and ... facilitating change than men" (p. xv). Overall, Book (2000) concluded, "Evidence is mounting that the style of leadership women offer is beneficial not only to employees but also to the bottom line" (p. xv).

Women have made important contributions to how we think about the way organizations can and should work. For example, women-run organizations often reflect a "web" structure (Helgesen, 1990a, 1990b), rather than a pyramid or typical hierarchical one.

Helgesen (1990a) reported that the women in business whom she had studied tended to disdain the hierarchical ladder and create webs rather than pyramids. In these webs, the leader is in the center of things, rather than at the top, which these women perceived as "a lonely and disconnected position" (p. 13). Webs allow everyone in the organization to be connected by invisible strands that emanate from the central goal or mission, and they value affiliation and win/win situations instead of intense competition and win/lose situations. In such a structure, "talent is nurtured and encouraged rather than commanded, ... a variety of interconnections exist, influence and persuasion take the place of giving orders, ... the lines of authority are less defined, [there is more dependence] upon a moral center, [and] compassion, empathy, inspiration, and direction" (p. 225) all play significant roles. Finally, webs allow the group to take full advantage of every person's talents and skills, permit a more effective exchange of information, and minimize conflicts that arise from misunderstanding or lack of communication.

This type of "connective leadership" (Lipman-Blumen, 1992) is endorsed as a style that "fits" with today's organizations. It incorporates networking, relationship building, empowerment, and mutual responsibilities between the leader and followers.

Leadership in this kind of organization encourages interdependence, increased involvement of all members of the group, communication, and consensus, all of which are needed in the chaotic world of today and tomorrow. Helgesen (1990a, 1992) asserted that women possess the skills, perspectives, and values needed to engage in this type of leadership. Indeed, in contrast to the Great Man Theory of leadership, which claims that some men are born leaders, Weddington (1991) asserted, "some leaders are born women." One would expect, therefore, that women would assume stronger positions of leadership as we progress in the 21st century.

COMBINING THE BEST OF "FEMALENESS" AND "MALENESS"

Schein (1989) cautioned us to be careful when talking about "feminine leadership" and said that the assumption that women lead differently than men is dangerous and perpetuates sex role stereotyping. She reported that research shows more differences within each sex than between the sexes, noting, "as individuals, executive women and men seem to be virtually identical psychologically, intellectually and emotionally" (Morrison, White, & Velsor as cited in Schein, 1989, p. 156). This author did suggest, however, that women might lead differently if our organizational systems were changed, and she urged America's corporate executives to restructure the work setting so that work and family are no longer separate but interface, a model similar to the one that exists in Norway and is quite successful. For example, if either parent needs to pick children up at school in the afternoon, the workday is structured to accommodate this "out of the office" responsibility.

In a work setting that values both career and family and that is more understanding of and willing to struggle with accommodating this interface, women would be likely to be more successful (Schein, 1989). In light of women's tendency to prefer "webs" to "pyramids" in the work setting and in other arenas (Helgesen, 1990a, 1990b) and the growing number of women-run businesses that reflect this organizational approach, we may, indeed, see the emergence of women as major players in making significant changes in our society, as Naisbitt and Aburdene (1990) suggested.

The new leadership paradigm that is emerging (and will continue to be needed in the complex, chaotic future) calls for individuals who facilitate interaction among leaders and followers, who empower followers, and who can successfully combine "maleness" and "femaleness" as an androgynous leader (Cann & Siegfried, 1990; Lipman-Blumen, 1992; Park, 1997; Schein, 1989). The androgynous leader blends dominance, assertiveness, and competitiveness—all of which are needed in a world where resources are increasingly limited—with concern for relationships, cooperativeness, and humanitarian values, which also are needed in a world characterized by chaos, uncertainty, and ambiguity. Table 6–2 suggests what women and men both need to do to be androgynous, and the next case study provided illustrates the different styles of a male and a female unit manager, as well as how each adopted characteristics of the other to enhance her/his effectiveness as a leader in the institution.

Women do think and act differently than men, and nurses have a perspective that is different from that of physicians. Instead of this being something about which we should apologize, however, or something women and nurses should try to change, it is something we should celebrate. The differences are something both men and women should exploit and use to benefit the increasingly diverse patients, families, and communities to whom we provide care. By combining the best of

TABLE 6-2 Becoming Androgynous

For women to be androgynous, they need to:

• Be powerful, forthright, and have a direct, visible impact on others.

• Be entrepreneurial.

• State their needs and refuse to back down.

• Recognize the equal importance of accomplishing the task and being concerned about the relationship.

• Build support systems with other women and take collective action.

• Be able to intellectualize and generalize.

• Deal directly with anger and blame, thereby rejecting feelings of suffering and victimization. Be invulnerable to destructive feedback.

• Talk and cry at the same time.

• Respond directly with "I" statements rather than "you" statements.

• Be analytical and systematic and share abstract models.

• Take more risks with power.

• See themselves as agents of change.

• Continue to be supportive and passionate, and become more autonomous and independent.

For men to be androgynous, they need to:

• Give evidence of how and why their lives are men's lives.

• Understand how men value women—as validators of masculinity, as a haven from the competitive male world, as the expressive partner in the relationship.

• Be aware of how physical and political power determine behavior.

• Openly express feelings of love, fear, anger, pain, joy, loneliness, and dependency.

• Personalize experience as opposed to relying on objectivity and rationality.

• Build support systems with other men, sharing competencies without competition, sharing feelings and needs.

• Learn how to fail at a task without feeling one has failed as a man.

• Value an identity that is not totally defined by work.

• Assert the right to work for self-fulfillment rather than to play the role of provider.

• Listen empathetically and actively without feeling responsible for problem solving.

• Enjoy friendships with both men and women.

"female leadership" and "male leadership," our visions can be more clearly articulated and better communicated. We can be more effective in guiding change and enhancing the abilities of followers. We can strengthen our organizations and improve patient care, and the nursing profession can become more powerful.

The humanitarian qualities that women leaders tend to possess need to be guarded carefully against erosion; however, the pragmatic orientations that male leaders tend to possess cannot be ignored. In an age when resources are increasingly scarce and competition reigns, organizations and professions must be focused, firm, bottom line–oriented, and realistic. In such a "pragmatic age" (Fuller, 1979), however,

Case Study

Natalie and Sean were nurse managers on different units of the local medical center. Both had qualified staff who respected their managers, and the patient care delivered on both units was considered by many in the institution to be exceptional. Natalie and Sean both participated regularly in the institution's management council, though Sean often was more assertive in offering solutions to problems being discussed and contributed more often to the critical conversations underway.

Natalie admired Sean's assertiveness, his willingness to offer an idea despite knowing it was not likely to be received very well, and his ability to remain objective even in highly charged situations. Sean, on the other hand, was impressed with Natalie's consistent concern for how proposed changes would affect and be received by staff, the network and support system she seemed to have created for herself and on which she called in difficult times, and her ability to energize her staff and the management council.

One day after a particularly difficult meeting, Sean and Natalie went to the coffee shop for coffee before returning to their respective units. They talked about the meeting, how the conversation evolved, the decisions that were made, and the contributions made by various participants, including each other. Each shared what they admired about the other's leadership skills and expressed a desire to "be more like the other" in some ways.

These colleagues, who were two of the most influential members of the management council, talked about how they could help each other. Sean agreed to use his comfort with being assertive to "open the door" for Natalie to speak more freely and perhaps disagree with or offer an alternative to what has been proposed, saying something like, "It looks like Natalie has some ideas swirling around in her head about this issue. Natalie, is there something you can share to help us think this through more effectively?" And Natalie agreed to "push" Sean to always consider how his ideas — though they may lead to an acceptable and quick solution — might be more effective if staff were involved in making decisions, saying something like, "Sean, your idea sounds quite reasonable, but what if we all asked our staffs to brainstorm about it before we go ahead and implement it? They may have an even better approach."

As a result of this dialogue and the willingness and concerted efforts of Sean (to take on more "female" leadership qualities) and Natalie (to incorporate more "male" leadership qualities), each of them grew as more effective managers and leaders. Their contributions to the management council were consistently valuable, and all members of that group looked to them to outline a vision for future directions, suggest ways to empower staff, and lead organizational change. The staff on each of their units grew professionally, and many of them were soon providing leadership, not only on their unit, but in the institution and in their specialty organizations and communities as well.

when any means may be used to reach the desired end (e.g., reducing standards to fill positions, failing to encourage self-care in patients so that they remain dependent, and cutting professional staff to make the bottom line look healthier), it is increasingly important that humanistic leadership be exercised!

> *Don't accept the dictates and little boxes that say, 'This is how the world operates.' You really have to push outside the hierarchy.* —Vera Martinez

STRATEGIES FOR WOMEN AND MEN TO BE SUCCESSFUL LEADERS IN THE FUTURE

In his initial examination of the trends that seemed to be shaping our lives, Naisbitt (1982) did not address the female/male phenomenon, suggesting, perhaps, that in

1982, women were not thought to be a significant force in shaping the future of our society. In subsequent writings (Naisbitt & Aburdene, 1990), however, the role of women became more prominent and even became the subject of a trends book in and of itself (Aburdene & Naisbitt, 1992).

Thus, we are increasingly aware of the significance women have in shaping the future of our world. We also are increasingly sensitive to the different perspectives women and men "bring to the table." What we also need to be fully aware of, however, are the strides being made by both genders to maintain their uniqueness while at the same time incorporating characteristics of the other.

According to Gordon (1991), "Women do not change the world by becoming more like men" (p. 15) and giving up the "female perspective" totally. Instead, they must work to "create a much needed sense of collaboration and community within the workplace" (p. 285) and other settings so that feminine values can be practiced alongside masculine values.

To become influential leaders and effective agents of social change, women—and men—will need to engage in individual and collective action. The following strategies may be helpful as women and men pursue leadership goals, particularly because many women—as they do approach leadership roles differently from men—lack self-confidence in that role (Farley, 1999):

- Participate fully in the mainstream of broad social and political activity, as well as in arenas of power and influence. Do not allow yourself to be isolated.
- Abandon your self-image and the public image of powerlessness and helplessness. Do not be naive about the realities of power and its uses.
- Refuse to align yourself with the culturally stereotypical female or male expectations. Do not let your need to achieve be sublimated to your need to nurture and serve, or vice versa.
- Continue to advance your education. The nurse influentials in Vance's (1977) study listed scholarship and intelligence as the most important attributes needed by nurse leaders of the future, qualities that are still seen as critically important (May, 2001).
- Do not allow yourself to be affected by the "impostor syndrome" (Harvey, 1985; *The impostor syndrome*, 1986), a phenomenon common to women (Goleman, 1985; Jacobs, 1985). Instead, both women and men must believe that they have achieved success because of their skills and talents, not because of some "fluke" or because of sheer luck.
- Develop collective strategies for action. Engage in teamwork and be willing to help others rather than distrusting them and seeing them as competitors, disaffiliating from each other, devaluing alliances, and seemingly wanting to "go it alone."
- Be politically and intellectually astute.
- Get involved in decision-making and policy-making boards.
- Be goal directed, and include "providing leadership to achieve a vision" among those goals.

- Take advantage of the positive leadership traits you possess. Acknowledge those strengths.
- Assure others of your competence by earning the right credentials and receiving competitive job offers and outside acclaim.
- Learn how to give and receive help from men or women without having those interactions become sexual encounters.
- Dress powerfully, not like someone of no importance.
- Take a visible seat at meetings and participate actively.
- Seek assignments to ensure that "the woman's (or man's) point of view" is represented.
- Seek mentor relationships or apprenticeships with others who have been successful in exercising leadership (May, 2001). Women may particularly want to seek other women as mentors.
- Be sure that others know of your accomplishments and achievements.
- Develop a positive sense of yourself and your abilities.
- Be supportive of others, but be careful not to take on their responsibilities.
- Develop your own support systems.
- Take a stand rather than "play it safe."
- Shape your world rather than just fit into it.
- Make your presence felt.
- Be proactive. Position and prepare yourself to take advantage of opportunities that present themselves or that you might create.
- Act based on power and choice, not based on fear.
- Learn confrontation skills and how to manage conflict effectively.
- Know yourself—your strengths, your vulnerabilities, your goals, and so on.
- Develop teamwork experiences for others (e.g., students, staff nurses).
- Take charge of your own destiny.

> *The best way to predict the future is to create it.*
> —*Yogi Berra*

CONCLUSION

In her examination of "The 100 Most Influential Women of All Time," Felder (1996) noted that these women—who were more likely to be writers and social reformers than scientists—have had a great and long-lasting "historical and cultural impact, have inspired us, and . . . have much to teach us about past and present culture, society, and selfhood" (pp. ix–x). She asserted the "indisputable significance of women's past, present, and future contributions to the world" (p. x).

Likewise, Schiff's (2005) analysis of nine women who changed modern America "influenced the political agenda [regarding segregation, child labor, reproductive rights, and other significant social issues] in creative, innovative ways" (p. xii). Thus, women need to take pride in the unique role they can play in providing leadership.

Women and men both need to hold onto the strength of their uniqueness, but at the same time, incorporate talents typically exhibited by the other. In other words, a movement toward more androgynous leadership and organizations that combine the benefits of hierarchies with those of "webs" may be most effective for the individuals in those groups or organizations, the individuals and communities they serve, and the professions they represent.

CRITICAL THINKING EXERCISES

Observe a female nurse and a male nurse in interaction with patients, physicians, and each other. What are the similarities between their communication and interpersonal styles? What particular differences do you notice regarding what seems to be important to each, what values each conveys in his or her communications and actions, how each approaches a problem or conflict, and so on? How do your observations compare with the differences discussed here?

_____

_____

Think about your own childhood and current situation. What were some of the "rules" by which you were expected to behave? Were those rules made explicit to you, or were they merely implied or suggested? What differences, if any, do you recall about how boys and girls behaved in grammar school and high school and what each group seemed to value? Do you think your experiences were fairly typical? If so, what can you conclude about how parents, schools, and the larger society socialize boys and girls into stereotypical roles? Also, discuss this with your colleagues who may be 10 to 20 years older or younger than you! Have we "come a long way, baby" in terms of a more androgynous approach to grammar school education, for example?

_____

_____

Select one of the women listed in Felder's (1996) book (e.g., Eleanor Roosevelt, Margaret Sanger, Harriet Tubman, Rosa Parks) and read a more extensive biography about her. To what extent did she reflect the characteristics of women leaders discussed in this chapter? To what extent did she also incorporate "masculine leadership" behaviors to be more androgynous? What strategies can you identify from this analysis that might help you be more effective as a leader?

_____

_____

Write a poem of 20 lines or less that conveys the essence of the strength of "feminine leadership" and that of "masculine leadership." Now read that poem out loud. Given all that you have read and thought about this topic and all the many things you could have said, what points were most significant to you that you absolutely had to include them in your 20 lines? Why do you think these points are so significant to you?

_____

References

Aburdene, P., & Naisbitt, J. (1992). *Megatrends for women.* New York: Villard Books.

American Association of University Women. (1992). *How schools shortchange girls. Executive summary.* Washington, DC: American Association of University Women.

Austin, N.K. (2002). The buzz about women leaders. *Leader to Leader, 26*(Fall), 56–60.

Babcock, L., & Laschever, S. (2003). *Women don't ask: Negotiation and the gender divide.* Princeton, NJ: Princeton University Press.

Book, E. W. (2000). *Why the best man for the job is a woman.* New York: Harper Business.

Brooks, A. (1983). For the woman: Strides and snags. *The New York Times,* October 16, 1983, p. 31.

Cann, A., & Siegfried, W. D. (1990). Gender stereotypes and dimensions of effective leader behavior. *Sex Roles, 23*(7/8), 413–419.

Farley, S. (1999). Leadership. In R.C. Swansburg & R.J. Swansburg (Eds.), *Introductory management and leadership for nurses: An interactive text* (2nd ed.) (pp. 456–478). Boston: Jones & Bartlett.

Felder, D. G. (1996). *The 100 most influential women of all time: A ranking past and present.* New York: Citadel Press.

Fuller, S. (1979). Humanistic leadership in a pragmatic age. *Nursing Outlook, 27*(12), 770–773.

Goleman, D. (1985). Feeling like a fake. *The Executive Female, 8*(5), 34–37.

Gordon, S. (1991). *Prisoners of men's dreams. Striking out for a new feminine future.* Boston: Little, Brown.

Grunwald, L. (1992). If women ran America. *Life, 15*(6), 36–46.

Harvey, J.C. (1985). *If I'm so successful, why do I feel like a fake? The impostor syndrome.* New York: Pocket Books.

Helgesen, S. (1990a). *The female advantage: Women's ways of leadership.* New York: Doubleday Currency.

Helgesen, S. (1990b). The pyramid and the web. *The New York Times Forum,* May 27, 1990, p. 13.

Helgesen, S. (1992). Feminism and nursing—"Feminine principles" of leadership: The perfect fit for nursing. *Revolution: The Journal of Nurse Empowerment, 2*(2), 50–57, 135.

The impostor syndrome. (1986). *Management Solutions, 31*(8), 18–19.

Jacobs, S. (1985). How businesswomen overcome a malady—"Impostor syndrome." *New England Business, 7*(E), 66–67.

Kellerman, B., & Rhode, D. L. (2006). Viable options: Rethinking women and leadership. In W. E. Rosenbach & R. L. Taylor (Eds.), *Contemporary issues in leadership* (6th ed.) (pp. 257–267). Boulder, CO: Westview Press.

Klenke, K. (1996). *Women and leadership: A contextual perspective.* New York: Springer.

Kram, K. E., & Hampton, M. M. (1998). When women lead. The visibility-vulnerability spiral. In E. B. Klein, F. Gabelnick, & P. Herr (Eds.), *The psychodynamics of leadership* (pp. 193–218). Madison, CT: Psychosocial Press.

Levenstein, A. (1981). Leadership and sex. *Supervisor Nurse, 12*(1), 15–16.

Lipman-Blumen, J. (1992). Connective leadership: Female leadership styles in the 21st century workplace. *Sociological Perspectives, 35*(1), 183–203.

Long, S. (1998). Discourse and corporate leadership. Transformation by or of the feminine? In E. B. Klein, F. Gabelnick, & P. Herr (Eds.), *The psychodynamics of leadership* (pp. 219–245). Madison, CT: Psychological Press.

Maccoby, M. (1981). *The leader: A new face for American management.* New York: Simon and Schuster.

May, L. K. (2001). *Leadership skills and attributes for Houston women in the 21st century.* Bellaire, TX: Greater Houston Women's Foundation.

Melia, J., & Lyttle, P. (1986). *Why Jenny can't lead: Understanding the male dominant system.* Saguache, CO: Communication Creativity.

Naisbitt, J. (1982). *Megatrends: Ten new directions transforming our lives.* New York: Warner Books.

Naisbitt, J., & Aburdene, P. (1990). *Megatrends 2000: Ten new directions for the 1990's.* New York: William Morrow.

Park, D. (1997). Androgynous leadership style: An integration rather than a polarization. *Leadership and Organization Development Journal, 18*(3), 166–171.

Robinson-Walker, C. (1999). *Women and leadership in health care: The journey to authenticity and power.* San Francisco: Jossey-Bass.

Rosener, J. (1990). Ways women lead. *Harvard Business Review, 68*(6), 19–24.

Schein, V. E. (1989). Would women lead differently? In W. E. Rosenbach & R. L. Taylor (Eds.), *Contemporary issues in leadership* (2nd ed.) (pp. 154–160). Boulder, CO: Westview Press.

Schiff, K. G. (2005). *Lighting the way: Nine women who changed modern America.* New York: Hyperion.

Sexes differ on military force. (1985). *Higher Education and National Affairs, 34*(23), 7.

Stivers, C. (1991). Why can't a woman be less like a man? Women's leadership dilemma. *Journal of Nursing Administration, 21*(5), 47–51.

Vance, C. N. (1977). *A group profile of contemporary influentials in American nursing.* Unpublished doctoral dissertation, Teachers College, Columbia University, New York.

Vance, C. N. (1979). Women leaders: Modern day heroines or social deviants? *Image, 11*(2), 37–41.

Weddington, S. (1991). Some leaders are born women (The Novello Lecture). Paper presented at the National League for Nursing Convention, Nashville, TN, June 11, 1991.

CHAPTER 7

Disequilibrium and Chaos: Challenging, Invigorating, and Growth-Producing

LEARNING OBJECTIVES
- Describe the process by which leaders and followers can thrive and grow despite the chaos of today's healthcare system.
- Describe how chaos and complexity science can propel individuals and organizations to accomplish goals.
- Analyze how nurse leaders can use the change process effectively in the realization of a vision.
- Formulate strategies that decrease resistance to change.
- Describe how purposeful introduction of conflict can generate change.

INTRODUCTION

Surviving the tumultuous "white water" of the current healthcare system—with its redesign and increased emphasis on cost containment—is a tremendous challenge for nurses and other healthcare providers, as well as for patients, families, communities, and organizations. Providers must create new systems, partner more effectively with one another and with patients, and work cohesively to provide cost-effective quality care and achieve desired patient outcomes. They also need to change the way they think about care and consider the patient's whole health status, not merely separate illness episodes. Patients must begin to become significant stakeholders in their own health.

115

As we move from the Scientific (or Newtonian) Age to the Relationship (or New Leadership) Age, nurses must incorporate a new perspective: that chaos is a good thing because it is what makes us evolve and grow. Nursing leaders need to be willing to make educated guesses, use their intuition, and be comfortable with uncertainty and ambiguity, rather than expecting to rely on formulas that a computer may generate from patient acuity codes. Nurses must take the time to develop leadership ability so that they can be the force that drives the profession's evolution and creates our preferred future.

As nurses, we can no longer remain as we are today. Instead, we must become comfortable with chaos and disequilibrium and adopt a new perspective on change. For example, Wheatley (2006, p.137) remembered listening to a geologist during a radio interview regarding his perspective on a huge hurricane in the Outer Banks. The interviewer asked what he expected to find after the hurricane. Instead of saying all of the negative findings one would expect, the geologist said: "I expect to find a new beach." In organizations, we also have to be willing to "find a new beach." We need to appreciate "how life is capable of so much change, so much newness," and "embrace this newness instead of trying to control it" (Wheatley, 2006, p. 139). We need to find time to use our intuition to solve problems, rather than focusing all of our energy on finding the parts that are not working and trying to fix them, as we so often do. By taking a new view of problems, we can identify "images, words or patterns that surface" (Wheatley, 2005; Wheatley, 2006, p. 141) that will help us focus on the whole and anticipate how growth and positive outcomes can be generated from the situation.

We must develop adaptive skills to manage conflict, the ability to delegate effectively to other healthcare workers, creativity to develop new caring strategies, maturity to recognize our lifelong learning needs, and the astuteness to position ourselves in arenas where significant decisions are being made. In other words, it is time to begin "walking the walk," rather than merely "talking the talk," and this requires leadership.

ADJUSTING TO THE LEADER ROLE AND THE PRACTICE OF LEADERSHIP

Nurses must acclimate themselves to feelings of uneasiness, ambiguity, and the unknown. By applying quantum theory principles (Malloch & Porter-O'Grady, 2005), we can realize that all systems work from the inside out, not from the top down or bottom up; and appreciate that relationship is as significant as control in maintaining effectiveness. Although systems cannot be predicted with certainty, we know that tension between stability and chaos creates change. The new leader, therefore, must do the following (Dreher, 1996):

- Stand on the edge of previous knowledge and ability.
- Transform problems into solutions.
- Be a part of a universe that never stands still.
- Realize that the ability to adapt to change is more important than being specialized in a field.
- Be able to help others resolve and grow from conflict.
- Focus more on cooperation than on competition.

Leadership is changing from a more individualized, unit-focused perspective to a participative focus. In fact, the Center for Creative Leadership recently examined how leadership is changing. Its report, *The Changing Nature of Leadership* (Martin, 2005), concludes that leaders must become more flexible and collaborative, be able to lead change and cross boundaries to build new relationships, and be willing to partner with others to shape the future. Findings from the study reported in this book indicate that skills such as resourcefulness, decisiveness, and doing "whatever it takes" that defined one as successful in 2002 have now been replaced by new skills like those mentioned previously.

> *Use the constant change around you as your opportunity to change people's perceptions of you, and to prove your skills and ability to contribute.*
> —Susan Rehwaldt and Mary Lou Higgerson

DEFINING CHAOS

Chaos, or extreme, unpredictable disorganization and surprise, is most apparent in the world today. Wheatley and Kellner-Rogers (1996) remind us that a "system maintains itself only if change is occurring somewhere in it all the time" (p. 33). So, one must view chaos or disorder as a means to survival. In other words, if there were no arguments or differences of opinion, the status quo would be maintained and there would be no individual growth. In addition, organizational survival would be threatened. The following questions were posed by Wheatley (2006, p. 73) to those who tend to believe that everything has to have a place and be labeled and filed away:

- Why would we stay locked in our belief that "truth" exists in objective form?
- Why would we stay locked in our belief that there is one way to do something, or one correct interpretation to a situation, when the universe welcomes diversity and seems to thrive on a plurality of meaning?
- Why would we avoid participation and worry only about its risks?
- Why would we resist the powerful visions and futures that emerge when we come together to co-create the world?
- Why would we ever choose rigidity or predictability when we have been invited to be part of the generative dance of life?

Questions such as these invite one to discard old ways and embrace new ideas like chaos theory. Many creative, motivated, and enthusiastic individuals thrive on chaos and are most successful in their personal and professional lives, despite the incredibly confusing climate in which they function. Others may become depressed and wallow in the disorder. For example, some nurses who are temporarily assigned to a different unit see that situation as an opportunity to expand their knowledge, skills, and networks. However, other nurses get angry with having to work on a different unit and may become so absorbed with that anger that they cannot rise to the assignment, barely maintain safety, and complain to anyone who will listen, including patients, their families, and nursing students. Is it this latter group of nurses' insecurities, fear of the unknown, or inability to deal with change that prevents them from turning what is seen as a bad situation into something positive? If situations such as these were to be seen as opportunities for learning new things, fear of the unknown could be minimized, and individuals would learn new skills and decision-making abilities. As a result, one would expect such individuals to grow more confident and increase their ability to survive the "chaos" associated with having to work on different units.

The way we perceive our situations in life, at work, and in our personal lives will greatly affect the outcome. Leaders see possibilities instead of adversities (Stoltz, 2000) and they know to keep "shuffling the cards" until visions are realized (Hader, 2005, p. 6). For example, conducting patient rounds where nurses share their approaches to caring for a patient allows new and experienced nurses to dialogue, learn a great deal from one another, and refocus the "negative" energy that may accompany new experiences. When everyone and everything can link together, systems form that create more possibilities for all. "This is why life organizes, why life seeks systems . . . so that more may flourish" (Wheatley & Kellner-Rogers, 1996, p. 19).

This perspective helps explain why nurses need to start leading as soon as they graduate and why they need to develop their leadership skills as they grow and evolve throughout their professional careers. The Robert Wood Johnson Foundation and the Institute for Healthcare Improvement (IHI) developed the *Transforming Care at the Bedside Initiative* to recognize the staff nurse as a leader in best practices of delivering healthcare (IHI, 2003). This is an excellent start, but each nurse must make a commitment to continue to develop her/his leadership ability.

The introduction to Michael Crichton's book, *Prey*, (2002), is entitled: Artificial Evolution in the 21st Century. In this piece, this physician author notes, "If we were to grasp the true nature—if we could comprehend the real meaning of evolution—then we would envision a world in which every living plant, insect, and animal species is changing at every instant, in response to every other living plant, insect, and animal. Whole populations of organisms are rising and falling, shifting and changing. This restless and perpetual change, as inexorable and unstoppable as the waves and tides, implies a world in which all human actions necessarily have uncertain effects. The total system we call the biosphere is so complicated that we cannot know in advance the consequences of anything that we do" (p. ix). Health care is similar, in that we cannot know in advance what is going to happen to each individual patient. In attempting to attain the most positive outcome for each patient, we need to manage multiple variables and be alert to the possible influence of variables we do not even know about.

Crichton further explained: "The fact that the biosphere responds unpredictably to our actions is not an argument for inaction. It is, however, a powerful argument for caution, and for adopting a tentative attitude toward all we believe, and all we do" (p. x). It is this tentative attitude that nurses need to assume so that when change occurs, they can be flexible and still succeed in attaining optimum patient outcomes. Last, Crichton said: "We are one of only three species on our planet that can claim to be self-aware [human beings, chimpanzees, and orangutans], yet self-delusion may be a more significant characteristic of our kind" (p. x). Nurses who are leaders do not decide themselves. Instead they attend to the realities and possibilities inherent in time of chaos and learn and grow as a result of the unanticipated occurrences that occur in our lives everyday.

CHAOS IN NURSING

From a Newtonian perspective, a leader is expected to help organizations adapt to change by establishing goals, obtaining commitment to the goals from employees at all levels in the bureaucracy, and decreasing uncertainty (Malloch & Porter-O'Grady, 2005). Such behaviors reflect the following assumptions (Wilson & Porter-O'Grady, 1999):

- If something works once, keep trying it.
- If employees' needs are identified, managers can manipulate them to improve the organization but not necessarily the employee.
- Large effects have large causes.
- Each employee should confine himself or herself to his or her specific job description.
- Given the organizational structure, one should know that lines of authority and information flow are similar.

One can see that this view emphasizes management, planning, and controlling, rather than leadership and empowering a group. The new leadership paradigm helps us realize that individuals are more effective leaders when they can keep their organization on the edge of confusion because it is only then that the whole organization can grow in a creative and productive fashion.

The uncertainty of healthcare flows from the quantum and chaotic nature of the world over time. We should, therefore, stop trying to plan every step and predict each happening. We must realize that we can never come close to knowing all there is to know about a topic, nor is it possible to plan every step. "The universe is no longer seen as made up of a multitude of objects, but as one indivisible dynamic whole with interrelated parts that can be understood only as a pattern of a cosmic process" (McDaniel, 1998, p. 343). Hence we have to accept that no matter how much we know about the world, there are far more questions than there are answers, and uncertainty is a natural part of our lives.

Nurses also have to realize that the lengthy "to-do" task lists they routinely develop at the beginning of a workday can be nothing more than skeletal frameworks because such lists cannot possibly encompass all that nurses will need to do that day. Being extremely task oriented and using a minute-to-minute structure to organize one's work must give way to critically thinking and constantly adapting as new problems and challenges arise. Because of the exceptional complexity of the nursing role today, organizational charts, time management lists, and critical pathways have served almost as survival techniques by giving some structure in a highly chaotic environment. Unfortunately, to-do lists and predictive pathways inhibit our ability to see things globally. Instead of trying to block out the chaos and unpredictability inherent in healthcare, nurses need to learn how to embrace it. McDaniel & Driebe (2005) recommend that groups such as nurses and other healthcare workers embrace complexity science in order to widen their leadership skills. One must embrace relationships with others and be aware that the order of life is based more on principles of emergence than on pre-determined order. Variables such as communication and cooperative relationships among individuals energize a system and help it be effective.

Nurses, however, also cannot simply "wait and see" how things evolve. Brown and Eisenhardt (1998) suggested a strategy, Competing on the Edge, to help manage chaos yet keep moving forward. This strategy consists of five key steps (p. 4):

- Improvisation
- Co-adaptation
- Regeneration
- Experimentation
- Time-pacing

The main premise of these authors is that, by attending to all five steps, individuals and organizations can obtain insight into what most likely will occur and, therefore, they can be positioned with the right resources to potentially succeed. Nurses can do this by hiring more diverse staff to work with the more diverse patient population, focusing on retaining current staff instead of recruiting new ones in order to regenerate the energy and passion of the staff, trying methods that do not require the same expensive resources that have been used in the past, and assisting staff in experimenting with new ideas that will help develop new practice models.

COMPLEXITY OF THE REGISTERED NURSE ROLE IN THE CURRENT HEALTHCARE SYSTEM

What seems to be a key to success in these ever-changing times is having the ability to appreciate the interrelationships among multiple variables. For example, when a new managed care system takes effect, several chronically ill patients may be forced to transfer to another primary care provider. When that happens, no patient–provider relationship exists, and all involved parties must begin all over again. In addition, it probably will take more time for the new provider to care for these complex patients, compared with the original provider, because he or she does not know the patient. The payer will have to pay for more visits, the patient has to worry about getting to the new office and building trust with the new provider, and the patient and provider will have to invest energy into starting a new relationship. The RN can be the consistent piece and assume the role of coordinating patients and providers so as to provide some type of consistency with the patient and family and the healthcare system. This type of case management is needed more than ever before to advocate for the maximum quality of patient care.

Complexity and collaboration are two sides of the same coin. —Kathleen Dracup

Many healthcare agencies and institutions have experienced change either through merging or acquisition. Nurse leaders can help avoid some of the problems that have accompanied such change (Seago, 1997, pp. 49–50):

- Minimize the number of major changes occurring simultaneously.
- Be proactive and network with the other healthcare workers when change is being planned.
- Be very involved in the day-to-day work of one's agency and remain cognizant of the challenges faced by all providers.
- Be held accountable for doing one's work well.
- Clearly define measures to evaluate patient outcomes.

FACILITATING LEADERSHIP IN CHAOS

Tonges (1997) suggests the following principles for succeeding where chaos reigns:

- Stay informed about the players in your work setting.
- Know and be guided by your values.
- Learn and use new technology.
- Accept and work with change.
- Renew yourself.

Neubauer (1998) agrees with these principles and recommends that people concentrate on renewing themselves, a process she defines as continuous self-assessment, being aware of one's own reactions, obtaining feedback, caring for oneself, and setting goals. Leaders also should call upon the diverse perspective of followers to brainstorm solutions and create the vision, focus on ongoing learning and the continued development of critical thinking skills, and communicate effectively. Further suggestions for providing strategic leadership in uncertain times are enumerated by McDaniel (1998, pp. 358–361):

- Stop planning and being preoccupied with order so that you can learn to cope with the unknowable.
- Move to the edge of chaos in order to find creative and new directions.
- Expect many people to be leaders because this will make for a vibrant organization.
- Allow for nurse autonomy so that people can learn to adapt and adjust to change in their own way.
- Improve the connections between colleagues because "the quality of connections between workers is more important than the quality of each individual" (p. 359).
- Do not allow people to say "That's not my job." Instead, teach them what other people are doing and help them appreciate that everyone is important if the vision is to become a reality.
- Assist peers to become "skilled at handling ambiguous issues, revealing differences, and generating new perspectives" (p. 360).
- Assist organizations and people to discover goals themselves.
- Work smarter, not necessarily harder.
- Provide for the emergence of new visions.

In his video, "Leadershift: Five Lessons for Leaders to Use in the 21st Century" Barker (1999) recommends the following:

- Focus on the future.
- Realize the nature of the change.
- Understand how systems operate.
- Reassess one's style of leadership to determine its impact on productivity.
- Build bridges to the future by developing a shared vision.

Barker asserts that leaders will assist people working in their teams to be 20 times more productive than if they were not working in a team. Barker also suggests that a dollar invested in a company with a vision will generate success approximately six times more than a competing company without a vision. It seems that if one can follow Barker's recommendations, it will assist a person to lead in chaos.

It is wise to realize that no matter how much energy is spent trying to lead through chaos, the stability one might long for is not really the solution at all because stability will only dampen the growth that occurs when some degree of chaos remains. Thus, each of us must become comfortable with constant change.

> *Nothing endures but change.* —Heraclitus

CHANGE

It has been said that the only permanent thing in society is change. As humans, one of the most pervasive and significant concepts affecting our lives is that of change—change that comes about through our own development and maturation, change that takes place as a result of our education and our interactions with others, change that is imposed on us from outside sources, and change that we impose on ourselves and others. If we are to cope effectively with change and use it to our advantage, we must be able to recognize when it occurs, when it needs to occur, how to facilitate it, how it can be blocked, and the impact various changes and change strategies have on individuals and groups.

Change is the making of something that is different from the way it was. It is an alteration; it results from differences and conflicts in a system, from information, or sometimes from unfulfilled needs. Change potentiates or allows the possibility of accomplishment of goals. It can be planned, or it may be an unexpected result of a decision or other event. Change can evolve over time, or it can be a spontaneous, revolutionary occurrence. Change in one's personal and professional life can involve a transition period, during which adjustment may be successful or not. No matter what the change, a true change does not affect only a single person; instead, it permeates the ambiance of a setting and triggers some type of change in anyone who comes in contact with the individual or setting that changed.

Belasco (1990) says organizations are similar to elephants in that they both learn through conditioning. He describes this phenomenon with the following illustration (p. 2): "Trainers shackle young elephants with heavy chains to deeply embedded stakes. In that way the elephant learns to stay in its place. Older elephants never try to leave even though they have the strength to pull the stake and move beyond. Their conditioning limits their movements with only a small metal bracelet around their foot—attached to nothing." Like powerful elephants, many individuals are bound by conditioned constraints. "We've always done it this way" is as limiting to an individual's progress as the chain around the elephant's foot.

It is time we move the nursing profession forward by listening to new ideas and trying new ways of doing things. We have to start "dancing" rather than feel chained to an invisible stake in the ground, and we need to start paving our own roads to our dreams. Many people often remark that they would change their lives dramatically if they could, and they say the change would focus more on gaining self-respect and increasing quality time with family and friends, rather than on gaining power and affluence.

Denhardt and Denhardt (2006) also speak to the dance of leadership. They assert that leadership can be perceived as being "drawn directly from the arts" (p.6) and of being an "intense textured interplay of space, time, and energy" (p. 6). These authors also differentiate leadership from management by saying leadership is all about "what energizes people," and to energize others a leader must try one thing and then another until a path reveals itself (p. 10). Additionally, "leadership is a way of working within a world of openness and change," whereas, "management is a way of working within a world of order and regulation" (p. 10).

It seems that many people are dissatisfied with their lives but do not know how to change. They have, in a sense, been conditioned to accept their lot in life and do not know how to move away from their routine—no matter how uncomfortable or dissatisfying that life has become. Perhaps by better understanding some principles of change (Box 7–1), we can be more willing to engage in it and change our lives.

THE LEADER AS A CHANGE AGENT

As nurses acquire new abilities and transform into leaders, they will demonstrate courage by involving others in clarifying the vision and making decisions about how to realize it. Decisions about quality of clinical outcomes, work content, and performance effectiveness of workers will be more readily incorporated if they are influenced

---

BOX 7-1 **Principles of Change**

- A change in one part affects other parts and other systems.
- People affected by the change should participate in making the change.
- People should be informed of the reasons for the change.
- Concrete and specific feedback about the process of change will enhance its acceptance.
- People need assistance in dealing with the effects of the change.
- People's suggestions and contributions about the implementation of change should be sought and incorporated.
- A change must be reinforced or the system will revert to its old practices.
- Conflict may occur at any step during the change process.
- The more compatible the new ideas are with one's values and needs, the more easily a change will be adopted.
- The more trust one has in the initiator of change, the more likely one is to support the change.
- One's past experience with change can profoundly affect one's willingness to support a new idea.

by nurses and not just the manager. Nurses are responsible for their own practice; thus, they should exercise leadership and direct that practice. The days of "my nurses are such good workers" and "I need one more RN for the Saturday eleven-to-seven shift, can't you do me a favor and work a double?" must come to an end. It is not the nurse manager's unit but the staff's. In fact, the "power" of the nurse manager will not be diminished—and may actually increase—when he or she empowers others to make change.

> *The secret to leadership is . . . to think of your position as an opportunity to serve, not as a trumpet call to self-importance.* —J. Donald Walters

Kouzes and Posner (1995) believe that leaders do not always seek the challenges and consequential ramifications of change that occur, but that these challenges seek the leaders. They also believe that challenge is the motivating milieu for excellence. They have found through their research that "ordinary" men and women are able to accomplish extraordinary feats, and those who function as leaders in the group realize they have skills they never knew they had, including the ability to manage change (p. 53).

An important skill for a leader to exercise when involved in change is that of coaching. This is the ability to facilitate others' understanding of themselves and their own abilities. It is the process by which one person (the coach—the leader) helps followers understand that answers to questions or solutions to problems lie within themselves. Being able to role model behaviors that assist individuals' adaptation to change is also helpful. Leaders who can help facilitate connections among followers should be successful in orchestrating a change. Dolci (2005) emphasizes this idea with his statement that "leadership focuses on flexibility, collaboration, crossing boundaries and collective leadership" (p. 4). This validates the importance of mentoring and coaching and confirms that the emergence of leaders is quite likely to result from such processes (Grossman, 2006). What nurses do in their lives everyday produces a certain type of wisdom, and this wisdom will assist nurses to lead others. By following what Kilburg (2006) calls "executive wisdom," the leader can help staff rise to their highest level of competency.

The new leadership is about forming relationships and connecting with others to challenge old, bureaucratic organizational structures and old ways of doing things. Such conventional assumptions about the use of teams (Ashmos, 1998) and the involvement of effective followers, as well as new perspectives on those assumptions, are outlined in Table 7-1.

The delay in committing to a decision allows followers or all those affected by the decision to discuss all issues fully and explore all possible options. Change requires giving up old behaviors so that new ones may be taken on, and it undoubtedly will cause conflict; however, if this conflict is addressed effectively, the new behaviors will be adopted and the ultimate outcome will be better. It is likely that as followers

TABLE 7-1 The Use of Teams—Working with Followers

CONVENTIONAL ASSUMPTIONS	NEW PERSPECTIVES
Followers are expected to commit to and accept decisions made by others.	Effective followers delay commitment to and acceptance of decisions until they have been able to assess their long- and short-term implications and their value in realizing the commonly held vision.
The role of followers in decision-making is to help gather necessary information.	Effective followers help the organization "unlearn" and then relearn.
Followers are valuable because they help create order in organizations.	Effective followers help create disorder so that groups and organizations continue to grow.
Followers enable execution of the organization's strategy.	Effective followers help decide the group's or organization's strategy.
Followers support and reinforce the hierarchy that is essential for goal achievement.	Effective followers reduce the hierarchy by questioning the effectiveness and efficiency of rigid structures.
All followers are guided by the organization's beliefs, more so than their own .	Effective followers challenge the group's or organization's beliefs.
Followers are empowered by leaders or managers.	Effective followers empower themselves.

Source: Adapted from: Ashmos, D. (1998). Building effective healthcare teams. In W.J. Duncan, P.M. Ginter, & L.E. Swayne (Eds.), *Handbook of healthcare management* (pp. 313–337). Malden, MA: Blackwell.

explore various options and points of view, turmoil in the group or organization will occur. Rather than being distressed by this turmoil, however, leaders are excited by it because it is exactly what the organization needs if change is to be successful. Teams of followers should be expected to cause continuous change in the group's or organization's strategy as they generate ideas for action and identify new directions. Reducing the existing hierarchy and challenging the group's or organization's belief system are necessary components to prevent an organization from maintaining the status quo. When an individual, group, community, or team is able to empower itself, effective leadership has occurred, positive change is likely, and the organization can grow tremendously. With this new perspective, the importance of developing self-directed teams of effective followers in any organization is made abundantly clear.

FACILITATING THE CHANGE PROCESS

Leaders are necessary to facilitate change. The environment must be ripe or made ripe. There must be a reason for the change to occur, and the players must be willing to try to change. The change must also yield growth—positive or negative. Such actions require that the leader be willing to think in new ways and try new approaches despite the barriers to change that they confront.

Knox and Irving (1997) studied nurse manager's ($N = 15$) perceptions of healthcare executives' behavior during organizational change and rank-ordered those perceptions from most common to least common (Table 7–2). The findings of this study reinforce the importance of effective communication, recognition of staff welfare as well as patient safety during a transition, and empowerment of staff to accomplish the processes necessary for the change to evolve. Such findings can be of great value to nurses who are attempting to facilitate change in their group or organization. Currie (2006) studied how nurse managers contribute greatly to strategic change in healthcare organizations and found that part of the success they garnered was due to their partnerships with agencies outside their own organization. Again, it is the relationships established between nurses and others that assist in making a difference and leading change (Nagelkerk, 2006).

TABLE 7-2 Results of Nurse Managers' Rankings of Healthcare Executives' Behavior During Change

RANKING	BEHAVIOR
1 (highest frequency)	Frequent communication of plans and progress during the transition
2	High visibility on work units during the organizational change
3	Verbalized commitment within the institution for the quality of patient care during the transition
4	Verbalized commitment within the institution for staff welfare during the transition
5	Presentation of rewards and recognition for staff performance during the transition
6	Empowerment of staff to accomplish changes for which they are responsible
7	Presentation of opportunities for staff to clarify issues in a nonthreatening environment
8	Follow-up on staff suggestions and questions related to the transition
9	Offers of support and assistance for problem solving during the transition
10 (lowest frequency)	Presentation of informational and educational programs before implementation

Source: Adapted from Knox, S., & Irving, J. (1997). Nurse managers' perceptions of healthcare executive behaviors during organizational change. *Journal of Nursing Administration* 27(11), 37.

There is no doubt that effective change requires leadership; however, both leaders and followers must be motivated and energized to implement positive changes and thrive in the chaos that will ensue. The Readiness-to-Change Quotient (Fig. 7–1 at end of chapter) is one way to stimulate nurses' thinking about how they can shape future changes in healthcare and how open they and their organization are to change (Mason & Leavitt, 1998). It can help each of us gain insight about how ready we and our organizations are for the changes confronted by healthcare today, awareness of such "readiness-to-change quotients" can help leaders wanting to implement a change.

THE PROCESS OF CHANGE

The current and predicted rate of change in society in general and in healthcare in particular is phenomenal. Such change requires professions, groups, and institutions to reassess their goals, structure, culture, and planning processes. Leaders are faced, therefore, with enormous challenges that are energy-consuming, but are also revitalizing and rewarding. Leaders must help others see the need for change, work with others to implement change, evaluate the effect of change, and participate in each stage of the change process. They also must understand what people experience as they go through change.

Perhaps one of the most useful theories to help us understand this phenomenon is that espoused by Lewin in 1951. He identified three phases of change:

1. *Unfreezing,* in which people are preparing for change
2. *Moving,* in which people have accepted the need for a change and actually engage in implementing the change
3. *Refreezing,* in which the new change is integrated into the system and becomes part of the new norm or culture

For example, a unit practicing primary nursing is experiencing turmoil related to staffing and reporting, as a result of the increased acuity of patients and decreased number of registered nurses (RNs). It becomes obvious that old assignment methods are no longer working and some unfreezing must occur. The staff and nurse manager engage in brainstorming activities and decide, after exploring many options, to institute a charge position for each shift. Once the new charge position is started, the unit enters Lewin's moving stage and works to refine the position and its duties to make it most effective. As the unit adjusts to and incorporates the new position, refreezing, or the integration of the position into daily work, occurs. This approach to change is congruent with the new leadership style because it is a dynamic process planned or facilitated by the leader and followers, but then allowed to evolve spontaneously and mesh into the system.

Whatever change theory one applies, it is important to realize that the stages of change are merely categories to help our thinking, not discreet steps that begin and end abruptly. In other words, change typically is not a clear-cut process that can be achieved by following a formula. Transformational change, as noted earlier, is an evolving process that tends to be the product of a group's vision over time, and revolutionary change follows no clear-cut formula. Perhaps nursing is in the process of a revolution. It appears we have moved through the unfreezing stage and are in the process of moving toward a more autonomous role in the healthcare arena. Advanced practice nursing is taking hold in every setting of healthcare delivery, and patient outcomes are beginning to validate the significance of our contributions. RNs and hiring institutions are realizing the need for continuing education as the staff nurse position becomes more and more integrated into the healthcare team structure. RNs and physicians are collaborating more than ever before, and patient outcomes are being tracked to identify both the nursing and medical interventions responsible for outcomes. As outcomes become publicized, our profession must move toward the refreezing or integration of change stage.

Perhaps the following "rules" for achieving change in an organization (Porter-O'Grady, 1998) will be helpful to nurse leaders during the unfreezing, moving, and refreezing phases of change:

- *Make no exceptions.* Everyone must engage in the change process.
- *Read the signs.* Be aware of all kinds of trends that are occurring, not just those related to healthcare. The leader must be prepared to design the future, not merely react to it.
- *Empower the center.* Involve those people who will be expected to implement and be most affected by the change in the process.
- *Construct new architecture.* Provide the supports people will need as they make the change and integrate new practices.
- *Evaluate, adjust, and evaluate again since "change never begins nor does it end."* "People don't start to change or stop changing. Change simply is!" (p. 1).

> *There is a certain relief in change, even though it is from bad to worse; as I have found in traveling in a stage-coach, that it is often a comfort to shift one's position and be bruised in a new place.* —Washington Irving

BARRIERS TO CHANGE

The captain of a ship steers the vessel from one port to another using carefully plotted coordinates. Why then does the ship veer off its course, sometimes miles off track of the destination? Why does the ship end up beached on a shoal not marked on the charts? Why does an iceberg cut up the ship? The answer to all these questions is that life is unpredictable, and captains must consider many other factors besides coordinates when navigating their ships. Nurse leaders must also consider multiple factors and anticipate potential problems when instituting changes.

Many factors can serve as barriers to change, including decreased resources, lack of support, resistance, poor communication mechanisms, or pressures to get the day-to-day work done. The more barriers there are to the change, the more effort will be needed to deal with those barriers and, consequently, the less energy will be available to institute the actual change.

DEALING WITH CONFLICT GENERATED BY CHANGE

Leaders work to implement changes that will have positive outcomes, but they also need to realize that there may be negative outcomes as well. Those seemingly negative outcomes, however, may actually be positive ones. One of the most common outcomes of change is *conflict*, something that historically has been viewed as negative but can be quite positive. The positive results of conflict are growth, an ability to accept that what was can no longer be, and collaboration, which builds healthy relationships.

In the new science of leadership, conflict can be an outcome of change or serve as an instigator of change and ultimately growth. To deal with the conflict generated, some goals may need to be abandoned, the vision may need to be altered, and an extraordinary amount of energy may need to be invested to help the group move through the change. The evolution of individuals, groups, and organizations experiencing the change, however, far surpasses the time and effort involved. Dreher (1996) reminds us that the Tao says we can develop better harmony by looking for it within us—by decreasing our anxiety and defensiveness in conflict. Using both the yin (patience, process, and empathy) and yang (courage and positive action), Taoism suggests the leader must balance opposites within herself or himself and be able to manage and grow from conflict.

Leaders must be confident, focused, and able to balance personal and professional goals to successfully orchestrate a change. This gives them the energy needed to take on the challenge of change. People must have a "clear perspective and life balance." In order to lead in the midst of change and chaos, it is necessary to have a clear vision and support from one's followers. Ultimately, it is better to choose to change and design one's own approach to change than to have a change imposed by some external force.

> *Tentative efforts lead to tentative outcomes. Therefore give yourself fully to your endeavors. Decide to construct your character through excellent actions and determine to pay the price of a worthy goal. The trials you encounter will introduce you to your strengths. Remain steadfast. . . .and one day you will build something that endures, something worthy of your potential.* —Epictetus (Roman teacher/philosopher)

It appears that many nurses use avoidance to manage conflict. While this may seem like a good approach initially, avoiding a conflict ultimately causes tension among team members and negatively influences the care environment (Kelly, 2006). An example that portrays the conflict of many nurses follows:

Conflict Management Case Study

Susan, RN, and her colleagues on a high acuity medical unit have extremely challenging patient assignments. Additionally, they are usually assigned new unlicensed assistive personnel (UAP) to assist them. Susan and the other RNs usually feel that it would be easier to do the work themselves since they have to spell out every detail to the UAP, and they hardly ever have any consistency with the UAPs. Generally there are different UAP assignments each day. Often, like today, the RNs have to orient a float RN who has his own separate patient assignment and who has been told by the supervisor to ask the staff RN for assistance with anything about which he feels uncomfortable. The staff RN has a new UAP to orient, another staff RN, not familiar with the unit's policies and staff, who is asking questions, and responsibility for an extremely challenging patient assignment. The staff RNs are likely to expend only so much

Continued

energy and accept this type of working condition only so many times before becoming angry and not willing to follow this patient assignment model any longer. Whether the nurses stay in this job or not depends greatly on how effectively the leader can help them manage the anger or conflict, create a new model of orienting float nurses, and, even more importantly, assist in retaining nurses so that there is less need for floating. Leaders must know how to deal with change and the conflict typically associated with it. It is important for the leader to assist the staff in developing champions to develop a new model of orientation/cross training RNs. Being confident that a change can be made and that the staff RNs can be responsible for creating a new way of thinking about floating will be paramount for success (Vivar, 2006). Some ideas to manage this case include the following:

• Create a champion among the staff who believes in the need for a change and who will guide the creation of a new orientation/cross-training policy.
• Brainstorm so that all staff RNs [those assigned to the unit and those who float to it on occasions] can participate in developing the new cross-training model.
• Obtain feedback regarding the change from other units, an objective party, and administration.
• Facilitate collaboration between representatives of the staff RN group and nursing administration to find a solution that incorporates both parties' perspectives and allows for a win-win outcome for all.
• Evaluate the effect of the change after piloting it.
• Incorporate findings from the pilot to revise the new practice policy.
• Periodically evaluate the effects of the new cross-training policy.
• Implement the new policy on a broader scale.

It is important to teach nurses how to be assertive and communicate their feelings and ideas. Since it is the nurses who are responsible for their patients' care, it stands to reason they should be part of planning how to best make patient assignments and how to most effectively orient new staff — permanent and temporary floats. By using the above-mentioned strategies, nurses can better manage conflict and facilitate change on their units.

CONCLUSION

There is no doubt that nurses are experiencing enormous change in their practice and the environments in which they practice. Although we may bemoan the fact that leaders cannot control or predict what will happen in these uncertain times, we need to think of this situation as a good thing because the chaos that exists can be used to promote extraordinary growth for the profession, the organization, and all individuals involved in it.

Leaders must have the ability to know when the strategies selected to realize a vision need to be altered, and they must surround themselves with a team of effective followers who bring diverse perspectives to the situation. Networking, partnering, and collaborating are skills with which nurses have been successful, and they need to draw on those skills to coach followers, help them identify their strengths and build their self-esteem, so that they can more effectively manage the many changes the profession now faces and will continue to face in the future.

Leaders should strive to make changes in educational programs to focus on learning more than on knowing, changes in incentives for bedside nurses that recognize their significant contributions and allow them to continue to develop their expertise in that role, and changes that create more opportunities for nurses to engage in collaborative efforts with their nurse colleagues and other healthcare workers. As we experience the chaos of the 21st century, it is even more important for nurses to lead and participate in change projects that reshape healthcare practices and policy. Groups, organizations, and professions that survive will be ones that encourage all members to think beyond what is currently possible and continuously participate in change.

READINESS-TO-CHANGE QUOTIENT
PART 1: HOW READY AM I?

1= DON'T KNOW; 2=STRONGLY DISAGREE; 3= DISAGREE; 4=AGREE; 5=STRONGLY AGREE

1. I know the current status of national and state healthcare reform legislation.   **3**
2. I'm aware of how trends changing the healthcare system will affect my practice.   **4**
3. My colleagues and I on my work unit have discussed healthcare reform and its implications for our practice and our roles.   **4**
4. I can influence the course of change in my workplace.   **4**
5. Some of the changes occurring in healthcare reform are consistent with nursing's interests and concerns.   **1**
6. I integrate into my practice a concern for continuity of care.   **5**
7. I'm greatly concerned about patients' satisfaction with the care my colleagues and I provide.   **5**
8. Patient education is a major focus of my practice.   **5**
9. I've played a significant role in developing a plan for improving patient care during the past six months.   **4**
10. I have a plan for my own professional development to enhance my role in a changing healthcare system.   **5**
11. I know what my state nurses' association is doing to influence health care reform.   **3**
12. I've communicated with one of my legislators about nursing practice issues affected by government policy.   **2**
13. I'm involved in community organizations, such as the school board, citizen action groups, or political parties that have an interest in healthcare reform.   **2**
14. I can use JCAHO standards (or those of another accrediting body) to argue for changes in my healthcare organization that will foster better patient care.   **4**
15. I can discuss the market forces affecting my healthcare organization and my practice.   **3**

TOTAL (add the above points)   **54**

FIGURE 7-1 • Readiness-to-Change Quotient

Source: Mason, D., & Leavitt, J. (1998). The revolution in healthcare: What's your readiness quotient? In E. C. Hein (Ed.). *Contemporary leadership behavior: Selected readings* (5th ed.) (pp. 452–454). Philadelphia: Lippincott.

PART 2: HOW READY IS MY ORGANIZATION?

(NOTE: If you work for a public health agency, school, or industry, you may need to translate some of the questions here to better fit your practice setting.)

1= DON'T KNOW; 2= STRONGLY DISAGREE; 3= DISAGREE; 4= AGREE; 5= STRONGLY AGREE

1. My organization provides programs or forums for discussion of changes and trends in healthcare delivery. _____4_____
2. Nursing administration has developed a strategic plan for transforming nursing practice in my organization. _____4_____
3. The staff in my organization is encouraged to be creative and to introduce innovations for improving patient care. _____4_____
4. Patient satisfaction data are regularly shared with the staff. _____5_____
5. Continuous quality improvement or total quality management approaches have been used to improve patient care within my organization. _____4_____
6. Nursing is involved in decision-making about staff mix. _____4_____
7. My organization has developed a plan for expanding ambulatory care or enhancing continuity of care. _____4_____
8. My organization belongs to a larger network of healthcare delivery systems (for example, hospitals, outpatient clinics, home care agencies). _____5_____
9. My organization is in good financial health. _____5_____
10. My organization uses or plans to use advanced practice nurses. _____5_____
11. My organization supports the staff's continuing education, reeducation, and advancement to help bring about changes needed in patient care. _____5_____
12. Nurses are included on all committees in my organization involved in policy development and strategic planning. _____4_____
13. The chief nurse officer in my organization has the authority. _____5_____
14. My organization supports collaborative, multidisciplinary team approaches to patient care. _____5_____
15. My organization is visibly marketing its centers of excellence to the community it serves. _____5_____

TOTAL (add the above points) _____68_____

Directions: Add the number values of your answers to the statements in "How Ready Am I?" (Part I), and mark on the horizontal axis of the scoring grid the point that corresponds to the total. Similarly, add the number values of your answers to the statements in "How Ready Is My Organization?" (Part II), and mark on the vertical axis of the grid the point corresponding to that total. Then find on the grid the point whose coordinates are your two scores.

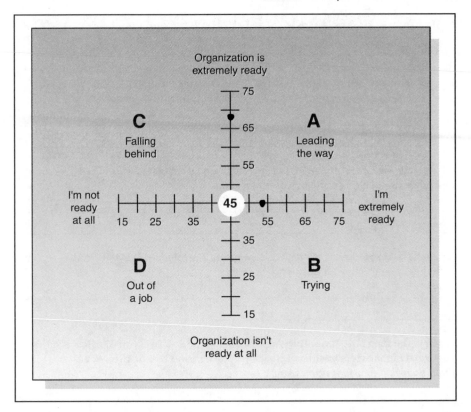

Here's what your score means: If your score places you in **quadrant A,** congratulations. You're "leading the way" and staying abreast of changes and trends in health care. And you work for an organization that's well positioned to thrive in a changing environment.

If you're in **quadrant B,** you're "trying," but either you don't know what's going on in your organization or your organization isn't doing much to inspire your confidence in its future. Ignorance is dangerous for both you and your organization. If you answered "I don't know" to many of the organization readiness questions, start to ask questions, read internal communications, and join committees that are planning the organization's future directions. If you didn't answer "I don't know" to most of those questions, your organiza-tion is in trouble—or will be soon. Given today's competitive environment, you'll need to take a hard look at whether you want to stay with your organization and have a strong enough commitment to help it move forward. You may want to assess how well other healthcare organizations in your area are poised for change and what opportunities they may offer.

If you scored in **quadrant C,** your organization may be reconsidering its commitment to you … you're "falling behind." Besides getting up to date with changes in your organiza-tion, you need to look beyond your workplace, at the big picture—what's happening in healthcare today and what will be happening tomorrow.

Finally, if you scored in **quadrant D,** you need to spend a great deal of time and energy learning about the changes in healthcare and looking for a healthier organization in your area. Chances are, you'll be "out of a job" unless your job happens to be at the only hospital or organization of its kind in the area, and is still experiencing a shortage of nurses.

Source: Mason, D. & Leavitt, J. (1998). The revolution in healthcare: What's your readiness quotient? In E.C. Hein (Ed.). *Contemporary leadership behavior: Selected readings* (5th ed.) (pp. 452–454). Philadelphia: Lippincott.

CRITICAL THINKING EXERCISES

Several authors assert that resistance to change grows out of fear. Talk to your nurse colleagues about why they have resisted change. Is the bottom-line reason that of fear? If so, what seems to be feared? If not, what is the bottom-line reason given?

_____

_____

What strategies have you used or experienced being used that have resulted in reduced resistance to and a successful outcome of change?

_____

_____

Given the "state of the art" of nursing, do we need a revolution? Do your nurse colleagues agree with your position?

_____

_____

Listen to the song "The Times They Are a-Changing" by Bob Dylan (1967). How is it that new expectations seem to emerge slowly yet still demand change? See Web site: *http://bobdylan.com/songs/times.html*

_____

_____

Listen to the song "Revolution" by the Beatles (Lennon & McCarthy, 1968). Why would some people prefer a quicker, revolutionary approach to change? See Web site: *http://www.bbgcarpet.com/revolutionbeatleslyrics.html*

_____

_____

Read an article about chaos in nursing in the journal *Complexity and Chaos in Nursing*. Describe how the new science of leadership correlates with how nurses practice leadership in a state of chaos.

_____

_____

View the movie *Witness* with Harrison Ford and Alexander Goodenauf. Amongst other story lines, this movie portrays how a group of people work effectively together to construct a building. What strategies can you take from this film to apply in your job to improve group work?

_____

_____

Use a personality inventory such as the Myers-Brigg to identify your individual personality style. Discuss how the results affect your ability to communicate and to resolve and grow from conflict. (http://www.personalitypathways.com/type_inventory)

_____

_____

References

Ashmos, D. (1998). Building effective healthcare teams. In W. J. Duncan, P. M. Ginter, & L. E. Swayne (Eds.), *Handbook of healthcare management* (pp. 313–337). Malden, MA: Blackwell.

Barker, J. (1999). *Facilitator's guide to Joel Barker's Leader-shift* video. St. Paul, MN: Star Thrower Distribution Corporation.

Belasco, J. (1990). *Teaching the elephant to dance: Empowering change in your organization.* New York: Crown.

Brown, S., & Eisenhardt, K. (1998). *Competing on the edge: Strategy as structured chaos.* Boston: Harvard Business School Press.

Crichton, M. (2002). *Prey.* New York: Harper Collins.

Currie, G. (2006). Reluctant but resourceful middle managers: The case of nurses in the NHS. *Journal of Nursing Management, 14,* 5–12.

Denhardt, R., & Denhardt, J. (2006). *The dance of leadership: The art of leading in business, government, and society.* Armonk, NY: M.E. Sharpe.

Dolci, J. (2005). The changing world of leadership. *Association Executive,* November/ December, 4.

Dreher, D. (1996). *The Tao of personal leadership.* New York: Harper Business.

Dylan, B. (1967). The times they are a-changing. *Bob's Dylan's Greatest Hits,* CBS Records Inc.

Grossman, S. (2006). *Mentoring in nursing: A dynamic and collaborative process.* New York: Springer.

Hader, R. (2005). Success is one leadership strategy away. *Nursing Management, 9,* 6.

Institute for Healthcare Improvement. (2003). Robert Wood Johnson Foundation *Transforming Care at The Bedside Initiative.* Accessed June 14, 2007, from *www.ihi.org/ IHI/Programs/strategicinitiatives/transforming*

Kelly, J. (2006). An overview of conflict. *Dimensions of Critical Care Nursing, 25*(2), 22–28.

Kilburg, R. (2006). *Executive wisdom: Coaching and the emergence of virtuous leaders.* Washington, DC: American Psychological Association.

Knox, S., & Irving, J. (1997). Nurse managers' perceptions of healthcare executive behaviors during organizational change. *Journal of Nursing Administration, 27*(11), 33–39.

Kouzes, J., & Posner, B. (1995). *The leadership challenge: How to keep getting extraordinary things done in organizations* (2nd ed.). San Francisco: Jossey-Bass.

Lennon, J., & McCartney, P. (1968). Revolution. *The Beatles, Past Masters,* EMI Records Ltd.

Lewin, K. (1951). *Field theory in social science: Selected theoretical papers.* New York: Harper & Row.

Malloch, K., & Porter-O'Grady, T. (2005). *The quantum leader: Applications for the new world of work.* Sudbury, MA: Jones and Bartlett Publishers.

Martin, A. (2005). The changing nature of leadership. Center for Creative Leadership. Accessed June 15, 2007, from *www.cd.org/leadership*

Mason, D., & Leavitt, J. (1998).The revolution in healthcare: What's your readiness quotient? In E.C. Hein (Ed.), *Contemporary leadership behavior: Selected readings* (5th ed.) (pp. 451–457). Philadelphia: Lippincott.

McDaniel, R. (1998). Strategic leadership: A view from quantum and chaos theories. In W. J. Duncan, P. Ginter, & L. Swayne (Eds.), *Handbook of healthcare management* (pp. 339–367). Malden, MA: Blackwell.

McDaniel, R., & Driebe, D. (Eds.) (2005). *Uncertainty and surprise in complex systems.* New York: Springer.

Nagelkerk, J. (2006). The process of change in healthcare organizations. *Clinical Nurse Specialist: The Journal for Advanced Nursing Practice, 20*(2), 93–94.

Neubauer, J. (1998). Thriving in chaos: Personal and career development. In E. C. Hein (Ed.), *Contemporary leadership behavior: Selected readings* (5th ed.) (pp. 247–258). Philadelphia: Lippincott.

Personal Pathways. (2006). What is your Myers-Brigg personality type? Accessed May 15, 2008, from *http://www:personalitypathways.com/type_inventory*

Porter-O'Grady, T. (1998). The seven basic rules for successful redesign. In E. C. Hein, (Ed.) *Contemporary leadership behavior: Selected readings* (5th ed.) (pp. 226–235). Philadelphia: Lippincott.

Seago, J. (1997). Five pitfalls of work redesign in acute care. *Nursing Management, 28*(10), 49–50.

Stoltz, P. (2000). *Adversity quotient at work.* New York: Morrow.

Tonges, M. (1997). The white water of change. *Nursing Management, 28*(10), 64–69, 70, 72.

Vivar, C. (2006). Putting conflict management into practice: A nursing case study. *Journal of Nursing Management, 14,* 201–206.

Waldrop, M. M. (1992). *Complexity: The emerging science at the edge of order and chaos.* New York: Touchstone.

Wheatley, M. (2005). *Finding our way: Leadership for an uncertain time.* San Francisco: Berrett-Koehler.

Wheatley, M. (2006). *Leadership and the new science: Discovering order in a chaotic world* (3rd ed.). San Francisco: Berrett-Koehler.

Wheatley, M., & Kellner-Rogers, M. (1996). *A simpler way.* San Francisco: Berrett-Koehler.

Wilson, C., & Porter-O'Grady, T. (1999). *The leadership revolution in health care: Advancing systems, igniting performance* (2nd ed.). Gaithersberg, MD: Aspen.

CHAPTER 8

Shaping a Preferred Future for Nursing

LEARNING OBJECTIVES
- Analyze how current societal healthcare trends can affect the future of nursing.
- Examine projections for the future that are likely to have an impact on the nursing profession and healthcare.
- Describe characteristics of leaders needed to shape a preferred future for nursing.
- Propose partnerships and collaborative relationships that can help nurse leaders shape a preferred future.
- Suggest strategies whereby nurses can create our own preferred future.

INTRODUCTION

Leaders in nursing have the responsibility to prepare today for tomorrow's challenges. Although we must be fully aware of our past so that we can learn from it, and fully aware of our present circumstance so that we can survive in it, it is perhaps more critical that we have some sense of the future, so that we can try to plan for it and shape it to our benefit. Leaders are responsible—through their vision, creativity, ability to facilitate change, and ability to manage and survive chaos—for articulating a preferred future for our profession and its practitioners, whether they be in clinical, administrative, educational, research, health policy, or other roles. Leaders, then, are responsible for helping create that preferred future.

Leaders can do this by creating bridges—interconnections between people that empower them and that change their focus from merely "doing their jobs" to having a larger purpose. Leaders must be integrators—seeing beyond the differences among various members of the group or team and using these divergent talents and perspectives to benefit the group. They must be diplomats—helping people get past their conflicts with one another and facilitate their working together. Leaders must be "cross-fertilizers"—bringing the best out of each group or individual and allowing that to be shared with the entire team. And they must be emotionally intelligent thinkers—those who can be creative and open to new possibilities that we have not thought of before. In essence, leaders foster collaboration among individuals and keep lines of communication open between all group members. It is also paramount that leaders encourage partnerships and collaborative teams in order to best secure our goals with the limited resources available. In the corporate world, there is a growing trend for "shared power models" in the work environment, and certainly the future will display increased numbers of mergers and acquisitions of industry conglomerates as well as healthcare groups (Bennis, 2007). Smith (2006) and Nedd (2006) both reinforce the importance of the care environment to generate strong individual and organizational performance by leaders and not necessarily with respect to individual variables such as age, experience, and tenure.

An orientation toward the future involves knowing current trends in our society and in the world; being cognizant of the social, political, economic, and organizational forces that create, influence, or are influenced by those trends; and speculating on the mutual interaction of these trends and forces with leadership needs (Ross, Wenzel, & Mitlyng, 2002). Leaders, however, cannot shape the future alone; they must engage others to achieve this goal. In the future it will be even more important to have an emphasis on cultivating followers. As Bennis (2007) says ". . . leaders do not exist in a vacuum . . . leadership in its simplest form is a tripod" consisting of "a leader or leaders, followers, and the common goal they want to achieve" (p. 3). Nursing leaders and followers must analyze scientific, technological, and healthcare trends and identify strategies to maximize the nurse's role in healthcare delivery.

Hillburn, McNulty, Jewett, and Wainwright (2006) and Matter (2006) urged nurses to use evidence-based practice protocols to participate in developing more reflective practice. They suggest that one of the ways to create the future is through using advances in science and technology. It is time for every individual nurse to get involved and make a difference in his or her practice area and in the profession as a whole, engaging in more reflective practice, which will [hopefully] improve morale and increase quality of care, as well as increase measurements such as patient satisfaction scores to reflect positively on nurses. These patient satisfaction survey assessment scores are a meaningful benchmark for institutions applying for or maintaining Magnet Status to recognize nursing contributions and reflect what nurses have identified as significant to maintaining their morale. Nurses must use their emotional intelligence, critical thinking, negotiating skill, and vision to create their future if we are to realize our preferred future.

PREDICTING THE FUTURE

When people talk about some of the things they expect to see in the future, it is often difficult not to laugh or roll one's eyes. Ideas that sounded like science fiction only a few years ago—Wikipedia [an online encyclopedia to which anyone can contribute], drugs individualized for each patient that attach to targeted receptor sites, battery-powered city cars that one uses for short distances and then parks to recharge, cars that are programmed to self-park, Styke connections via computer for global communication, and vacuum robotics—are very real in today's world. Ideas considered "way out," unreal, or unbelievable when they were first proposed are now common. The world is changing dramatically, the "good-old days" are gone forever, and the new "good-old days" are happening now. In healthcare, multiple trends are shaping a new future: the change to palliative care instead of hospice, addressing nursing staff and faculty shortage, and a need for a better way to manage healthcare financially. Just like several of the trends Naisbitt (noted in 1982) predicted that eventually became true, publications such as *Futurescan: Health Trends and Implications 2005–2010* (American College of Healthcare Executives, 2005) cite multiple predictions that imply some big changes for healthcare. Nursing leaders need to be aware of these trends, so the profession will be influenced positively and be a leading force in creating the future of healthcare system(s), not merely reacting and adapting to the impact of those changes.

> *There is only one direction for a leader: FORWARD.*
> —*Advertisement*

Kouzes and Posner (1995) recommend that we think of the future as a time for great things and that, in most instances, things will be improved. These authors surveyed leaders about the future and found that terms such as "foresight," "focus," "forecasts," "future scenarios," "perspectives," and "points of view" are common in discussions of visions of the future. It is important, however, that leaders be able to translate these global terms into detailed descriptors as much as possible when sharing the vision, so that followers can better understand what the vision represents and more fully participate in making it become a reality.

Obviously, there is no crystal ball, but there are methods that futurists can and do use to try to determine future happenings. Leaders must know a particular area well, understand how certain occurrences in this area were started and have evolved, and be knowledgeable about how patterns of related happenings might affect the area currently and in the future. This kind of information will assist the leader in knowing how and where to notice trends and determine if they are indicators of future patterns. Aburdeen (2005) reminded us to use past occurrences as we attempt to predict future ones. By examining these past trends and how they affected the world, we will be more prepared to anticipate consequences of the new trends and not be surprised.

Futurists recommend that leaders read what is new and predicted for the future, review the histories of significant developments, maintain a global perspective as to new issues and economical growth, and review information from sources like the Census Bureau and the Bureau of Labor Statistics. Every individual and every profession or group needs some context within which successful plans for the future can be made, and resources such as these help a leader create that context.

Four kinds of futures are addressed in the literature (Valiga, 1994):

1. The *probable future* is what is likely to occur if things continue as they are and no changes are made.
2. The *possible future* is what can occur if some changes are made in the current state of affairs.
3. The *plausible future* is what is likely to occur when specific efforts are made to accomplish goals.
4. The *preferred future* is what we would like to see happen.

Using this framework is a good way to brainstorm about the future. Small groups of nurses can create various scenarios that can increase our ability to visualize what different futures might be like and strategize how we can create the future we want for nursing. This might occur in a retreat setting where nurses engage in strategic vision planning, or it can begin to happen at staff meetings or during discussions over coffee.

By analyzing changes in societal values, public policies, and individuals' behaviors that are significant to the future of health, rather than dwelling merely on medical break-throughs, nurses can significantly influence the general welfare of humanity. For example, if society does not deal with poverty and illiteracy, both of which are related to illness, more people will use hospital emergency departments for their basic healthcare and increase the costs, less of an emphasis will be on health promotion and disease preven-tion, and the poor will be likely to have more illness complications. If nurses become involved in developing health policy that mandates health promotion for the unin-sured, impoverished, and illiterate, the people of the world are likely to have a greatly improved future.

> *Leadership is a process rather than an event. We don't always know how, when, or what we will lead. Each of us wants our life to stand for something. Being able to have an impact—to make a difference —is perhaps the biggest benefit of being a leader.*
>
> —Sarah Weddington

Nurses can make strong contributions in improving healthcare in multiple areas. By educating the public, providing testimony for changes in healthcare policy, providing wellness care to the poor and underserved, and speaking out about issues or injustices in one's workplace, nurses could significantly change the quality of life for many, as well as enhance cost savings and higher-quality health.

Most nurses would probably agree that the preferred future depicts a healthier, more educated population. Health promotion will reign, and wellness-focused health centers will populate the country and outnumber disease management clinics. Nurses, as leaders of health, must propel their visions forward and begin thinking in a future-forward frame, so that they can have more input into how the future will transpire.

Nurses in every aspect of care have the power, for example, to spearhead a massive anti-obesity campaign by educating all people about its negative impact on health. Who better than nurses to teach the population how to manage health, prevent illness, reduce complications of illness, and choose health resources?

Molitor (1998) reminded us to be aware of possible "wild cards," such as meteor strikes on earth, volcanic eruptions, or some other inconceivable events that could "throw quite a monkey wrench" into our best laid plans. We also need to realize that things no one had dreamed or thought to be so significant, such as individuals wanting to learn how to fly jumbo jets but not how to take off or land them, can have a significant influence on future developments. This uncertainty and unpredictability is exactly what we in nursing need—something to make us think! Today's new science of leadership makes us more open to the unknown becoming a reality and to accepting that the future holds endless possibilities for us. Despite this unpredictability, however, we must attempt to shape the future at least to some extent because "foresight enhances abilities to capitalize upon opportunities, decrease adversities, gain lead time for responding, and assert leadership in trying to manage change" (Molitor, 1998, p. 59).

The future does not just happen. We dream about it and shape it to some extent every day. Whenever a change is proposed, even if it is so small it will affect only one individual or one part of an organization, that change influences the future and can contribute to the growth of the organization or profession. Change of any type ultimately will have ramifications for any number of people.

> *There are three kinds of people: those who make things happen; those who watch things happen; and those who wonder what happened.* —Anonymous

An example from clinical practice may help illustrate this notion of interdependence and how a change can have a "ripple effect." A nurse in the cardiothoracic intensive care unit draws on research data and suggests that every nurse use the forced warm air blanket instead of the fluid-filled blanket to rewarm postoperative patients. The nurse implements this change for his or her own patients and monitors those patients' rewarming times, frequency of cardiac dysrhythmias, cost, and electrolyte balance. Consistent with reported research findings, this nurse finds that rewarming times are shorter, dysrhythmias are less frequent, electrolyte imbalances are reduced, and the cost of care is less. As a result of this change, this nurse's idea becomes a hospital-wide protocol. This nurse then disseminates his or her findings in a publication and is invited to address critical care nurses at a regional conference. The nurse's findings are validated at other institutions, and eventually a state-of-the-art postoperative rewarming standard of care is accepted. This is an example of how one idea, tested by one nurse, then acted on and followed through by other nurses, can generate a significant difference for patients and have a positive impact economically.

Perhaps more nurses need to advocate "killing sacred cows," not always sticking to a plan, and an "if-it-ain't-broke, break-it" philosophy. Such "radical" thinking allows more participation in developing a vision that is exciting, creating a future that is challenging, and creating new opportunities.

Today only about 20% of healthcare is delivered in the inpatient setting (as compared to 1980, when about 83% of the care was inpatient) and, in 1983, the average length of stay was 6 days (whereas today it is 2 days) (Bureau of Labor Statistics, 2005). Nurses continue to be the largest healthcare occupation with 2.4 million full-time RNs employed in the United States and a predicted 27% increase of more RN positions by 2014 (U. S. Department of Labor, 2007). It is important to be aware of the work being done by nursing workforce centers and the new initiatives in education, policy, service, and health services research they support (Cleary & Rice, 2005). The growing diversity of our population, aging baby boomers, technological advances, the genome model, and palliative care movement are trends that have had an impact on healthcare and will continue to influence the role of the nurse.

GENERAL PREDICTIONS ABOUT THE FUTURE

It is difficult not to be slightly pessimistic when considering some of the predictions about the future: global warming with its concurrent ecological collapse, nuclear or biological warfare, terrorism, increased violence, economic demise, and infectious diseases that are resistant to antibiotic therapy. Such predictions also can serve to challenge us to plan proactively to minimize these possibilities and their negative effects. They can promote enthusiasm about countering these trends, for example, by developing super antibiotics, connecting to alien civilizations, increasing the quality of life and life span, benefiting from our ability to map all 80,000 genes in human DNA, strengthening the total world infrastructure, and using solar power and other renewable energy sources.

> *If there is no struggle, there is no progress.*
> —*Frederick Douglass*

Advancements in consumer electronics will assist in greater communication, easier access to services, at-home jobs, less traveling time, increased leisure time, and new education avenues. Just for a moment, think about this possibility: all roads and cars are removed from the earth; the old roads are made into moving sidewalks where one steps on and, with a handheld apparatus, controls the direction and speed of one's trip. Just think of the decrease in trauma that would result if there were no automobile accidents. The reality is that most people still have cars, and traffic jams and accidents still exist. We can still envision, however, a preferred future in which energy is clean and conserved, and more travelers use super-fast rail systems, mini-battery charged city cars, and suborbital space travel. Changes such as these will affect global trade, influence how people interact with one another, how they spend their time, and possibly assist people in living a more productive life.

In addition to changes such as these, dramatic changes in family structures and population demographics will continue to occur. The family is no longer the primary social unit. There are more single parent families, grandparent families, and blended families than ever before. The U.S. population is approximately 301,139,947. Approximately 20% of the people in the United States are less than 14 years old, 67% between the ages of 15 and 64 years, and 13% more than 65 years of age. In addition, 82% are white, 13% are black, 4% are Asian, and less than 1% are other (CIA World Factbook, 2007).

The U.S. population currently makes up 4.7% of the world population, but it will make up only 4% of the world population in 25 years. Thus, America is not growing in population size the way many other countries are growing. There will be fewer young people in America, and the United States will have less of a voice regarding national and global issues. Currently, the median age in the United States is 36.6 years and the life expectancy is 75.15 for men and 80.97 for women. Of today's United States population 12.6% is at least 65 years old, and 20% of the population is expected to be at least 65 years by 2030; thus it is accurate to say a large portion of the healthcare business is and will continue to be caring for older adults (CIA World Factbook, 2007).

Approximately 24% of residents die in nursing homes or die shortly after a transfer to an acute care hospital from a nursing home (Strumpf, Tuch, Stillman, Parrish, & Morrison, 2004). In 2007 more people were reaching advanced old age (i.e., 85 years), and approximately one half of individuals who reach age 65 can expect to live at least an additional 20 years. Lunney, Lynn, and Hogan (2002) suggest that besides the 7% of older adults who experience sudden death, most of the other 93% of older adults have a spiraling down of their health and are challenged to manage multiple chronic illnesses before death. In projecting future healthcare needs of a growing older population, there is evidence they will experience some period of functional decline before death, even if they are healthier as older adults (Lubitz, Cai, Kramarow, & Lentzner, 2003).

Of the expected additional 13 years of life expectancy for people in good health at age 70, an average of 5.3 years will be spent in functional decline resulting from chronic illness, and an average 0.7 years will be spent in institutional long-term care. Deaths from chronic illnesses occur primarily in older adults: 83% from cardiovascular disease, 70% from cancer, and 88% from cerebral vascular accident (Arias & Smith, 2003). Because of the increase in the elderly population and the decrease in the younger population, the United States may give more priority to issues affecting the old versus those issues influencing the young. Diversity of the U.S. population will continue, and by 2010 fewer than 50% of U.S. citizens are expected to be of European descent (Molitor, 1998). With the increased number of retirees and decreased number of workers, the Social Security system is expected to be insolvent by 2030, or sooner, if measures are not put into place to safeguard the system. Ethical considerations for caring for the elderly, critically ill individuals with multiple-organ disease, the disabled, and those found to have genetic defects also will be more prevalent and force us to explore new alternatives to providing care for the very ill and dying. There will continue to be a paradigm change of providing palliative care to people with advanced chronic illnesses, as well as to the terminally ill.

PREDICTIONS ABOUT THE FUTURE OF HEALTHCARE

Healthcare costs in the United States were approximately $2 trillion in 2005, equaling 16% of the gross domestic product (GDP) and an average of $6,700 per person (*www.nchc.org/facts/cost*, 2006). It is expected that a conservative prediction for future healthcare costs in 2015 is $4 trillion. In 2006, employer health insurance costs rose by 7.7%, with the annual premium for single coverage averaging $4,200 and $11,500 for a family of four. Currently 47 million Americans are uninsured. It is no wonder, then, that cost is a major issue in healthcare today. In 2006, drug companies ranked as the third most profitable industry after commercial banks, and mining and crude oil production. Recently some organizations have started to import their members' drug prescriptions from Canada to attempt to decrease costs, hospitals send x-rays to India to be interpreted, and people have elective surgeries in countries other than the United States to save costs.

The issue of quality of healthcare is receiving long-awaited attention, and cost-effective outcome-measured healthcare has become an expectation. The American Nurses Association has responded by developing nursing-sensitive quality indicators that, if implemented in acute care settings and home care, can help nursing claim a significant leadership role in healthcare (Gallagher & Rowell, 2003). The emphasis on the quality of services provided at a reasonable cost has many benefits, such as more educated consumers; certification for healthcare providers; choice of healthcare provider (e.g., nurse practitioner, nurse anesthetist, nurse midwife, physician); more health partnerships; more independence for nurses and other nonphysician providers; telehealth; an outcomes-driven system; and, of course, improved care for patients, families, and communities. The emphasis on quality and the measurement of outcomes require that all healthcare professionals be accountable and responsible for providing competent interventions that generate positive patient outcomes. An example is described by Robert and Sebastian (2006) regarding implementation of a Tele-Intensivist Program through which improved patient safety and quality was demonstrated when computer physician-order entry, evidence-based hospital referrals, and intensive care unit (ICU) physician staffing were implemented. Another good example of how nurses were able to improve care significantly was the integration of a nurse-driven system for communicating reliable outcome information (Johnson, Hallsey, Meredith, & Warden, 2006).

In the future, healthcare will focus increasingly on the prevention of illness and the promotion of health, and more care will be provided in short-stay units, urgent-care centers, subacute facilities, and homes. Except for some very rural providers, most healthcare agencies are now affiliated with a large corporation, and healthcare has moved from independent, freestanding agencies to integrated networks that focus not only on primary or tertiary care but also on the entire continuum of healthcare delivery. It is expected that all healthcare agencies will continue to develop affiliations with other hospitals, homecare agencies, rehabilitation centers, subacute-care facilities, community centers, long-term care facilities, and laboratories, as well as develop satellite centers in the community to provide primary and secondary care to neighborhoods. Hospitals will no longer deal merely with health restoration but with health promotion and maintenance as well. In fact, policies are in place today where nonsmokers with a normal body mass index (BMI) can get reductions on their healthcare insurance premiums. Multiple possibilities will be beneficial in the future such as anti-aging antidotes, medications that decrease insulin resistance prior to even being diagnosed with diabetes mellitus, anti-obesity remedies, and drugs that can decrease lipid accumulation that are already being used. New techniques in diagnostic technology and genetic research are expected to move us from a "diagnose-and-treat" scenario (once symptoms are manifested) to a "predict-and-manage–in-a-proactive-fashion" scenario (even before symptoms are evident) that would include things like gene therapy to create new peripheral vessels for extremities.

Computerization will continue to allow all providers to access the patient's record, regardless of location, and patients/consumers will be able to access their records freely. Multidisciplinary teams involving physicians, nurses, social workers, physical therapists, psychologists, occupational therapists, and other providers we cannot even envision today will follow evidence-based protocols to deliver quality care to patients, and they will be delivering that care in the patient's home or community, including schools, malls, workplaces, satellite health centers, and other access points. These differences between the current healthcare delivery system and what integrated delivery systems (IDSs) of the future will be like are summarized in Table 8–1.

PREDICTIONS ABOUT THE FUTURE OF NURSING

Nursing shortages and patient safety are two of the most significant issues facing nursing in the future. One must consider, then, how the following predictions will influence

TABLE 8-1 Characteristics of the Past/Traditional and Future Healthcare Systems

Past/Traditional Healthcare System	Future Healthcare System
Episodic, fragmented	Continuous, coordinated
Individualized plan of care	Critical pathways
Sickness-focused	Health promotion- and disease prevention-focused
Insurance coverage	Managed care organizations
Inpatient care	Ambulatory and community-based care
Hospital as profit center	Hospital as cost center
Specialist physicians	Primary care practitioners
Independent solo physicians	Multispecialty group practice
Physician-dominated care	Nonphysician care providers
Fee-for-service payments	Predetermined capitated fee payments
Heavily regulated environment	Increasingly competitive environment
Provider-oriented	Consumer-oriented
Presumption of high quality	Documented quality

Source: Adapted from Buerhaus, P. (1998). Creating a new place in a competitive market: The value of nursing care. In E. C. Hein (Ed.), *Contemporary leadership behavior: Selected readings* (5th ed.) (p. 424). Philadelphia: Lippincott.

these issues. There are 26,000 unfilled RN positions in hospitals and 123,000 unfilled RN positions in nursing homes (JCAHO, 2003). In addition, openings for approximately 1 million RN positions are predicted for 2010 (Bureau of Labor Statistics, 2005). The U. S. Department of Health and Human Services forecasts a need for 7.5 full-time equivalent (FTE) RNs per thousand population in 2020, which is increased from 7 FTE RNs per thousand population in 2000 (*www.bhpr.hrsa.gov*). It seems there must be different ways to deliver nursing care so the predicted shortage will not mitigate our ability to provide safe and high-quality patient care.

Many elements of the chaos in healthcare, such as downsizing of healthcare institutions, changing from an illness to a wellness perspective, moving from private physician–dominated providers to multidisciplinary systems, and the use of capitated payment systems, all have had an impact on nursing. In addition, many demographic changes, such as the increasing elderly population, fatherless families, ethnic diversity, homelessness, and underprivileged people needing healthcare in their communities, provide increased opportunities for delivering care outside the hospital.

The nursing workforce itself needs more nurses who practice autonomously, use evidence-based nursing interventions that generate positive patient outcomes, are respected as experts in certain areas of patient care, provide input to the development of health policy, and participate fully on multidisciplinary healthcare teams. Both registered nurses (RNs) and advanced practice registered nurses (APRNs) *must* be accountable for patient outcomes and eliminate old ways of thinking, such as, "A nurse reports to the physician and merely needs to notify the physician about a change or document a finding about a patient in the patient record." Instead, if we are to create a preferred future for nursing, nurses must be responsible for identifying problems and seeing them through to a positive patient outcome. The future of the profession depends on nurses following through, taking responsibility, and documenting the outcomes of their research-based interventions. Only then will we truly be able to "sit at the table" with our colleagues from other healthcare disciplines and be recognized for contributing significantly to quality and cost-effective care. As stated earlier, nurses must become involved not only in predicting our future, but in creating the future we prefer. If we agree with Bennis (2007) that change fosters beginnings and not endings, and if we agree that the healthcare system is in chaos, then now is the time for nurses to create the future that will benefit patients, communities, and our profession by best utilizing all that nursing has to offer.

High technology, including patient monitoring systems, computerized medication administration, interactive computer communication, and computerized patient data storage, is a good example of how nursing can benefit from change. Technological advances such as those just mentioned maximize the potential for nurses to spend more time with patients, allow more independent clinical judgments, provide immediate communication with other members of the healthcare team, and help nurses manage patient data for quick retrieval when analyzing patient outcomes. Technology, therefore, should not be thought of as an enemy, but as an ally because it helps nurses be more autonomous. An example of this is distance education for nurses. Several models of educating nurses via Blackboard® modalities have been successfully instituted around the world and demonstrate how attitudinal, technical, and structural barriers were overcome, so that more nurses could become educated on a variety of topics (Lewis & Farrell, 2005).

The passing of the Balanced Budget Act of 1997, mandating direct payment to nurse practitioners, has had an impact on the future of advanced practice nursing (*www.healthlaw.org/bba.html*). However, nursing leaders must be certain to collaborate with the Medicare Commission to develop healthcare policy that allows this third-party payment to continue and be expanded. In fact, to shape a preferred future for nursing, all nurses should be involved with developing health policy, networking with legislators and political groups, and spearheading changes in the delivery of healthcare to consumers. Such action will enable nurses to influence necessary changes in healthcare that will improve the profession's image as a competent and powerful contributor to the health of the American people.

No longer can nurses focus solely on their particular unit or specialty area. Today's nurses cannot expect to work for the same employer throughout their careers, nor can they expect to do the same thing in nursing throughout their careers. They must be aware of the larger arena of healthcare, continue their education, and remain flexible. Nurses also will do well to focus on measuring nursing care outcomes, being attuned to cost effectiveness, ensuring high-quality nursing interventions, participating in ethical debates, providing access to healthcare for all, working collaboratively with one another and with other healthcare professionals, increasing our educational preparation standards, and being a vital voice in healthcare policy making. A good example of integrating nurse sensitive outcomes with the assistance of performance and workload indicators to justify nurse staffing ratios is explained by Griffin and Swan (2006).

> *Quality is never an accident; it is always the result of intelligent effort.* —*John Ruskin*

Nurses must take responsibility for shaping the future of the nursing profession, as well as for shaping their own careers. By studying patterns of change, being aware of important trends in one's specific area of nursing, keeping abreast of general healthcare literature, and talking to others involved in healthcare, nurses will be able to deal more effectively with the unexpected that the future is bound to bring.

All nurses need to be knowledgeable about multiple views of issues facing healthcare, nursing education, and the nursing profession, as well as to be flexible and capable of making a decision when the need arises. For example, a staff nurse directs the care of patients; reviews; and, in many instances, determines or coordinates what transpires between the healthcare team and each patient. In addition, he or she plays a negotiator role regarding what the patient should receive, what type of services, and when. The nurse also oversees ancillary workers, builds consensus in order to successfully implement patients' plans of care, takes risks in demanding patient safety and high-quality care be given, and empowers patients and other staff to speak up and be counted among those who will make a difference. Nurses need to be knowledgeable about the healthcare delivery system in which they work, as well as about the newest knowledge on which their practice is based.

It is important to realize that no single individual can determine what the future will be, but nurses can shape their own future by being cognizant of multiple possibilities and open to trying new, and even radical, changes. We cannot sit back passively and accept everything the future hands us; instead, we must create a preferred future of nursing. How can we do that? The following discussion is intended to help nurses become more effective in increasing their own ability to shape a preferred future for the profession and for healthcare.

Approaches to Shaping a Preferred Future for Nursing

Nursing education must prepare graduates who have the ability to participate as full partners in healthcare delivery and shape health policy. Nursing curricula should emphasize patient safety, patient education, health promotion, rehabilitation, self-care, alternative methods of healing, and palliative care while maintaining the concern for acute and tertiary care. Both accreditation bodies in nursing, the National League of Nursing Accrediting Commission (NLNAC) and the Commission on Collegiate Nursing Education (CCNE), recommend that nursing educators, along with nurse executives and clinicians in practice settings, shape practice. All curricula should include, at appropriate levels, case management, healthcare policy, research, quality indicators, outcome measures, financial management, legislative advocacy, and management of data. The notion of lifelong learning for all nurses to maintain competency must also be continually addressed, perhaps through mandatory continuing education or certification.

> *You don't have to be brilliant to be a good leader. But you do have to understand other people—how they feel, what makes them tick, and the best way to influence them.* —John Luther

Nurses also must clearly define what they do and communicate it to the public so that consumers will be able to understand the role of the RN and APRN. Malloch and Porter-O'Grady (2005) recommended that nurses expand their roles to work as consultants to the public, patient or professional specialty groups, healthcare equipment or pharmaceutical corporations, daycare centers, or any group interested in health. These exemplary entrepreneurs in nursing say that the skills of the staff nurse, grounded in practice and framed by the discipline of nursing, more than adequately prepare the nurse to take on the expanding demand of the consultant's role. In the future, more nurses who are competent in their specific area will be expected to serve as consultants, thereby increasing the public's knowledge of what nurses do.

The nurse leader must go further than identifying that there is a need for change and assisting others to be a part of the evolution of this change. Rather, nurse leaders need to promote new practice models (e.g., primary care clinics adjoined to emergency departments) in order to best maximize the use of the expensive resources and conserve costs. Another idea that could greatly assist with making the future of healthcare brighter, is to develop programs that allow older adults to stay in their own or family homes for a longer period of time before going to a long-term care facility. These changes in care delivery would positively affect healthcare even in the midst of a nursing shortage, high patient acuity, and escalating healthcare costs. Also, nurses can help each other visualize that many traditional nursing activities could become a part of the patient's own care process. Families and patients can be instrumental in decreasing costs and increasing quality of healthcare. This new paradigm drastically changes what nurses will be doing in the future. The uncertainty that exists at present regarding this paradigm change provides nurses with an opportunity to create and "test" new care models that increase accountability of patients and families for their own health. At the same time, nurse leaders must be sure nurses are involved in hospital initiatives regarding work flow, physical plant changes, and communication-related issues since these areas are highly related to patient safety problems (Thompson, Navarra, & Antonson, 2005). An example of how collaborating nurses and physicians decrease medication errors using safe practices is described by Rogers, Alper, Brunelle, et al (2006).

There is and will continue to be a need for "nursing support positions such as staff development coordinator and clinical nurse specialist and staff resource person to meet learning and socialization needs of inexperienced staff in increasingly complex clinical settings" (Russell & Scoble, 2003, p. 406). These positions could greatly influence inexperienced and new staff and assist with improving nursing retention in tertiary care centers.

Mathena (2002) recommends nurse managers have strong leadership skills to assist staff in adapting to the multiple mergers of healthcare organizations that are and will continue to occur. She cites the need for leaders to have "visioning, interdisciplinary team building, workload complexity analysis, work process analysis, stakeholder analysis and interactive planning skills" (p. 138) in order to maximize success. Her research identified communication skills as the most highly needed skill for nurse managers, and findings led this researcher to recommend education in financial and technical skill management for nurses.

All nurses have a professional responsibility to be involved in nursing organizations that are actively working to create a preferred future for the profession. Sigma Theta Tau International (STTI) and other organizations (e.g., the American Association of Critical Care Nurses and the Emergency Nurses Association) have committed to creating a positive future by offering leadership institutes, helping members expand their networks through the Internet or newsletters, and offering recognition through awards and citations as a way to motivate nurses to work at their highest possible level. Whether one is working at the local or chapter level as a committee member or officer, serving on a board of directors, working on an international committee, or reviewing manuscripts for an organization's journal, one is working to advance the future of nursing and shaping that future. Senge, Scharmer, Jaworski, and Flowers (2004) remind us that the ultimate focus for the future is to lead in a just and human way and advocate for all.

Research must be conducted to determine the extent to which research-based protocols are implemented along with the cost-effectiveness of the patient outcomes.

Nursing science must continue to be developed, so that nurses can provide care that will increase positive healthcare outcomes (Naylor, 2003). Additionally with electronic healthcare records and computerized physician order entry, more cost-effective and efficient practices will be facilitated.

Nurses must study the effectiveness of what we do and provide leadership regarding the nursing aspect of multidisciplinary research. We must continue to study the health-care practices of various groups, as well as patient responses to specific interventions. Such patient responses might include pain management, understanding of one's health status, stress level, and ability to perform self-care in order to maintain or enhance function. In other words, nurses must measure the effect of nursing care and not merely describe problems that exist in healthcare. Dissemination of results should be done in publications and presentations, including those that are multidisciplinary in nature and those accessed by the public. There must be a commitment to using research results as a basis for practice, and being involved in the conduct of research must be integral to every nurse's ongoing practice.

As noted earlier, the chaotic world of today needs more than just a few leaders at the top. Leadership is not a position but a process and a role that everyone can and must assume at some point in time. Staub (1996) suggests we look for leaders at all levels of society in all types of organizations, and he suggested such people are the ones who are comfortable with "fuzzy logic" and "approximations" (p. xv). Consider the light switch, which turns a light on or off, and a dimmer switch, which allows a light to vary in degrees of brightness. According to Staub (1996, p. xv), the dimmer switch, which can be compared to fuzzy logic or approximations, "allows for a greater range of response and therefore flexibility to the requirements of the environment. . . . So too, in real life, [where] the range of options can be extended to many more iterations between the two fixed positions of off or on, right or wrong, black or white. In approaching the challenge of our complex world, it is important to remember that while white matters and black matters, where it really counts is in gray matter(s)." Thus, leaders who will help shape a preferred future for nursing will benefit from the use of "fuzzy logic."

In essence, everyone has something to offer; there is a place on the team where each person can make important contributions. Perhaps if the strengths of all individuals were appreciated, and they were empowered, members of a team would develop the self-confidence to do their very best and make significant contributions to shaping a preferred future. This attitude of people working hard, feeling good about themselves, and having their contributions acknowledged can significantly affect the accomplishment of a once seemingly distant vision.

> *The reward of a thing well done, is to have done it.*
> —*Ralph Waldo Emerson*

Partnering implies teamwork, with every member being equal and all connecting horizontally, or via a web structure (Helgesen, 1990), rather than vertically or via a hierarchical structure. Using principles of partnership such as equity, accountability, and ownership, each member contributes a unique set of talents to achieve the common goal (e.g., quality patient care), each partner is patient centered, and no one tells another partner what to do or when to do it. Indeed, the healthcare system of tomorrow will not support the old type of authoritative behavior; instead, it will expect each person to own his or her part and do his or her job with excellence. Such a paradigm supports collaboration, dialogue, patient participation, freedom of expression, and empowerment, all of which are crucial to success. Nurses must take pride in the responsibility they have to monitor patients and provide health surveillance in all healthcare settings. We must take pride in the leadership we provide as case coordinators and the role we play in "holding the system together." This is what nurses do, and it is our unique contribution to healthcare. With the increase in equal partnering, nursing has a new frontier to pursue and new roles to assume.

CHARACTERISTICS OF NURSE LEADERS NEEDED TO CREATE A PREFERRED FUTURE FOR NURSING

Leaders of tomorrow must be transformational ones—people who can propel a vision, recruit the new generation of nurses, empower followers to work enthusiastically to realize a vision, meet change "head-on" and grow from it, exploit conflict to ensure people are thinking in different ways, and keep harmful stress at a minimum for themselves and the organization. They must be designers, teachers, and stewards (Senge, 2006): *designers* assist in developing the vision; *teachers* help followers develop the skills and gain the knowledge to work toward making the vision a reality; and *stewards* act as spokespersons for the group, keep the group focused on the vision, and facilitate the long-term growth of all followers.

Leaders have ideas about what the future can bring and what it could be like, but they do not just sit around and wait for things to happen. In fact, Bennis (2007), who has interviewed multiple leaders and identified common talents they possessed, concludes that exemplary leaders have six skill competencies that define them as leaders:

- Create a sense of mission
- Motivate followers to work with them on the mission
- Develop a social ambience for their followers
- Create trust and optimism
- Develop others to lead
- Obtain results

Leaders for the future take action, engage in self-evaluation, seek feedback from colleagues, set goals and periodically evaluate progress in meeting them, advance their own knowledge, and try new things (Valiga, 1994). Being able to envision the future and create a sense of vision separates leaders from others. Accepting the challenge of leading is a decision each of us must make. When we accept that challenge, we also accept responsibility for shaping a preferred future for nursing. We may be more successful in shaping a preferred future if we incorporate the following guidelines (Kouzes & Posner, 1995, p. 99):

- Do not wait.
- Have credibility . . . Be honest, be an inspiration, maintain competence, and be forward-looking.

- Have your head in the clouds but your feet on the ground . . . Always be thinking of possibilities but also stay grounded in reality.
- Share values.
- Accept that you cannot do it alone.
- Remember that leadership is everyone's business.

As long as one has a vision, articulates it clearly, enlists others to help make it a reality, is aware of factors that influence it, and is able to keep the vision on course, one really is a leader and is shaping a preferred future. It is much more exciting to help determine what the future will be than to merely react to it as it happens around us. True wisdom and true leadership come from learning from the past, enjoying and growing in the present, preparing for the future, and creating the future.

> *Never give up your credibility by saying, 'This may be a dumb question, but . . .'* —Elizabeth Tegues

Phenomenon of Leadership: What Is New and Should You Change Your Practice?

Everyone knows there are as many definitions of leadership as there are books on this topic. We must continue to review the literature on leadership and continually integrate new ideas and findings into our practice in order to grow personally and strengthen our profession. Since no formula for the leadership skills is needed in the future and because leadership is a dynamic phenomenon, we must be prepared to exercise different leadership skills as the future unfolds. We lead based on what has been successful in the past and what we learn from others (through reading, listening to presentations, observing or studying others, etc.). The following case study illustrates how nurse practitioners made significant differences in their practice by collaborating daily on a communication board.

Case Study

At a college health clinic, the nurse practitioners are seeing several patients complaining of pruritis from a rash randomly scattered on their legs. The lesions are isolated to the lower extremities, and the nurses soon determine that it appears to be poison ivy. Upon discussion with one another, they realize that the patients include many athletes from the track team that participated in a tournament presently going on in a nearby state. When more details are shared among the nurse practitioners, it is determined that the method of transmission is by droplets from running through puddles on the dirt road leading to the competition field. None of the students remember having direct exposure to poison ivy or any plants. One of the nurse practitioners calls the university where the tournament took place and shares the findings collected regarding the multiple cases of contact dermatitis resembling poison ivy. Representatives from the hosting university recall the grounds had recently had some pruning in preparation for the tournament and determine that there could very well have been clippings of poison ivy that have blown into the puddles. It is most reasonable to conclude, therefore, that as students run through these puddles, they are infected via the droplets.

The nurse practitioners identified a pattern, realizing there was a correlation with being at the tournament university and contracting poison ivy, communicated their findings with each other and the host university, and recommended that action be taken to prevent other athletes and bystanders from further exposure during the ongoing tournament. After seeing the positive outcomes of this experience, the nurse practitioners decided to institute the daily use of a whiteboard inside their office to document high frequency or unusual diagnoses they see in the clinic.

This whiteboard collaborative communication board has come to be a most helpful method of assisting with diagnosing. Because these nurse practitioners cared enough to "get to the bottom" of the poison ivy epidemic, they were able to make a difference. Likewise, the practitioners have been very successful in recognizing community-acquired methicillin-resistant-*Staphlococcus aureus* in wounds, identifying a scabies infected group of students, educating the wrestling team regarding impetigo, and other problems sooner than had occurred when they saw patients in isolation of each other and did not communicate as effectively.

This example of a common situation illustrates how nurses in any practice setting can choose to exercise leadership. Assimilating similar assessment data, detecting patterns, and finding commonalities between the data helped these nurse practitioners make a difference in the care they provided. These nurses were empowered to take the time and make a difference because they cared enough to discuss their intuitive thoughts. Nurses have much to share and can lead others in providing improved care to patients if they use their leadership competencies.

CONCLUSION

The world around us is changing dramatically, and the role of the nurse will continue to expand and evolve. In light of this, nurses must decide how we want the role to evolve and then plan to make that happen. It would seem that all nurses can embrace the vision of providing quality healthcare to anyone in need. What we need to do now is work collaboratively to make this vision a reality. We must think critically and communicate effectively with our equal partners on the healthcare team to determine the interventions that will result in the highest quality of patient care.

Leadership must be everybody's business. Apathy, doing only what is written in one's job description, retorting "I am only a nurse" or "That is not my job," failing to continue to learn, letting others make decisions for us, or continuing to assume a subservient role will not serve nurses well in the evolving healthcare system, and it will not help us create a preferred future for nursing. Every nurse must stand up for a cause, bridge a gap, network with others, and do what needs to be done to move our profession forward toward *the future we want.*

CRITICAL THINKING EXERCISES

Imagine that it is the year 2015 and you are about to be interviewed by an international nursing journal about the significant difference you have made to the nursing profession. What would you talk about? What significant differences have you made? How will you respond when the interviewer asks what you plan to do in the next 5 years to continue to make a difference?

_____

_____

Draw a picture of your vision of the future role of the nurse in your current area of employment. What could you do to make this vision a reality? Share your ideas with your nurse manager or colleagues.

_____

_____

Identify four positive and four negative events related to your nursing career or during your education as a nursing student that you have experienced in the past. Describe why each may have happened. Review the positive ones and determine a pattern, and review the negative ones to see if a pattern emerges there. What can you learn from this analysis that could help you shape your own professional future?

_____

_____

Given the predictions about the future in general, the future of healthcare, and the future of nursing, what kinds of nurse leaders will the profession need to shape a preferred future? Are these same qualities needed today? Why or why not? How will globalization affect these predictions?

_____

_____

Informally interview a variety of people (e.g., children, an older adult, a healthcare provider, nurse colleagues, a new college graduate) about the future of our society, our world, the healthcare system, and nursing. Ask them what they think things will be like in the year 2015 and beyond. Also, ask them what they think we need to do now to achieve the positive things they envision and avoid the negative things they think could happen. Are the views of nurses different from those of other groups? Are there differences in the views of nurses from different cultures?

_____

_____

References

Aburdeen, P. (2005). *Megatrends, 2010*. Charlottesville, VA: Hampton Roads.

American College of Healthcare Executives. (2005). *Future scan: Health trends and implications 2005–2010*. New York: Health Administration Press.

Arias, E., & Smith, B. (2003). Deaths and death rates for the 10 leading causes of death in specified age groups. U.S. preliminary 2001. *National Vital Statistics Reports, 2003, 51*(5), 26.

Bennis, W. (2007).The challenges of leadership in the modern world. *American Psychologist, 62*(1), 2–5.

Bezold, C. (1996). Your health in 2010: Four scenarios. *The Futurist, 30*(5), 35–39.

Bezold, C., & Mayer, E. (Eds.). (1996). *Future care responding to the demand for change*. New York: Faulkner & Gray.

Buerhaus, P. (1998). Creating a new place in a competitive market: The value of nursing care. In E. C. Hein (Ed.), *Contemporary leadership behavior: Selected readings* (5th ed.) (pp. 422–431). Philadelphia: Lippincott.

Bureau of Labor Statistics. (2005). U.S. Department of Labor, Occupational outlook handbook, 2005. Accessed June, 2007, from *http://www.blls.gov*

CIA World Factbook. (2007). Accessed June 5, 2007, from *http://ww.cia.gov*

Cleary, B., & Rice, R. (Eds.). (2005). *Nursing workforce development: Strategic state initiatives*. New York: Springer.

Gallagher, R., & Rowell, P. (2003). Claiming the future of nursing through nursing and sensitive quality indicators. *Nursing Administration Quarterly, 27*(4), 273–284.

Griffin, K., & Swan, B. (2006). Linking nursing workload and performance indicators in ambulatory care. *Nursing Economic$, 24*(1), 41–44.

Helgesen, S. (1990). *The female advantage: Women's ways of leadership*. New York: Doubleday Currency.

Hillburn, K., McNulty, J., Jewett, L., & Wainwright, K. (2006). Build upon strengths and leadership practices using EBP. *Nursing Management, 37*(11), 15–16.

Johnson, K., Hallsey, D., Meredith, R., & Warden, E. (2006). A nurse-driven system for improving patient quality outcomes. *Journal of Nursing Care Quality, 21*(2), 168–175.

JCAHO (Joint Commission on Accreditation of Healthcare Organizations). (2003). Quick stats on nursing shortage. Accessed June 15, 2007, from *http://www.JCAHO.org/ news+room/press+kits/quick+statistics+on+the+nursing+shortage.htm*

Kouzes, J., & Posner, B. (1995). *The leadership challenge: How to keep getting extraordinary things done in organizations* (2nd ed.). San Francisco: Jossey-Bass.

Lewis, J., & Farrell, M. (2005). Distance education: A strategy for leadership development. *Nursing Education Perspectives, 26*(6), 362–367.

Lubitz, J., Cai, L., Kramarow, E., & Lentzner, H. (2003). Health, life expectancy, and health care spending among the elderly. *New England Journal of Medicine, 349*(11), 1048–1055.

Lunney, J. R., Lynn, J., & Hogan, C. (2002). Profiles of older Medicare decedents. *Journal of American Geriatric Society, 50*(6) 1108–1112.

Malloch, K., & Porter-O'Grady, T. (2005). *The quantum leader: Applications for the new world of work.* Sudbury, MA: Jones and Bartlett Publishers.

Mathena, K. (2002). Nurse manager leadership skills. *Journal of Nursing Administration, 32*(3), 136–142.

Matter, S. (2006). Empower nurses with evidence-based knowledge. *Nursing Management, 37*(12), 34–37.

Molitor, G. (1998). Trends and forecasts for the new millennium. *The Futurist, 32*(6), 53–59.

Naisbitt, J. (1982). *Megatrends: Ten new directions transforming our lives.* New York: Warner Books.

Naylor, M. (2003). Nursing intervention research and quality of care: Influencing the future of healthcare. *Nursing Research, 52* (6), 380–385.

Nedd, N. (2006). Perceptions of empowerment and intent to stay. *Nursing Economics, 24*(1), 13–19.

Robert, A., & Sebastian, M. (2006). The future is now: Implementation of a tele-intensivist program. *Journal of Nursing Administration, 36*(1), 49–54.

Rogers, G., Alper, E., Brunelle, D., Federico, F., Fenn, C., Leape, L., et al. (2006). Reconciling medications at admission: Safe practice recommendations and implementation strategies. *Joint Commission Journal on Quality & Patient Safety, 31*(1), 37–50.

Ross, A., Wenzel, F., & Mitlyng, W. (2002). *Leadership for the future: Core competency in healthcare.* Chicago: Health Administration Press.

Russell, G., & Scoble, K. (2003). Vision 2020, Part 2. Profile of the future nurse leader. *Journal of Nursing Administration, 33*(7/8), 404–409.

Senge, P. (2006). *The fifth discipline: The art and practice of the learning organization* (2nd ed.). New York: Doubleday.

Senge, P., Scharmer, C., Jaworski, J., & Flowers, B. (2004). *Presence.* New York: Currency Doubleday.

Smith, A. (2006). Managing people or places. *Nursing Economic$, 23*(1), 45–46.

Staub, R. (1996). *The heart of leadership: Twelve practices of courageous leaders.* Provo, UT: Executive Excellence.

Strumpf, N. E., Tuch, H., Stillman, D., Parrish, P., & Morrison, N. (2004) Implementing palliative care in the nursing home. *Annals of Long Term Care, 12*(11), 35–41.

Thompson, P., Navarra, M. B., & Antonson, N. (2005). Patient safety: The four domains of nursing leadership. *Nursing Economic$, 23*(5), 331–332.

United States Department of Labor. (2006). *Health care occupations.* Accessed June 7, 2007, from *www.bls.gov*

Valiga, T. (1994). Leadership for the future. *Holistic Nursing Practice, 9*(1), 83–90.

CHAPTER 9

Developing as a Leader Throughout One's Career

LEARNING OBJECTIVES
- Describe ways in which individuals can develop as leaders.
- Describe the characteristics of an environment that facilitates the development of leadership skills in self and others.
- Relate the concept of empowerment to the development of leaders.
- Analyze the process of mentoring as it relates to the development of leaders.
- Propose a personal plan for leadership development that attends to empowerment, mentoring, role modeling, networking, self-assessment, and continued renewal.

INTRODUCTION

One of the early leadership theories, the Great Man Theory, espoused that leaders were individuals who had been born into the "right" family at the "right" time. This theory has been challenged over the years as being far from useful in understanding the multifaceted nature of leadership. Indeed, there is now widespread agreement that leaders are made, not born. The question remains as to how an individual can be "made" into a leader.

Individuals who are acknowledged as leaders do not simply declare that they will be leaders and expect that others will accept such a declaration. In addition, success in one role (e.g., faculty member) does not guarantee success in a leadership role (e.g., dean) (Gmelch, 2000). Instead, as demonstrated in our own profession (Houser & Player, 2004, 2007), individuals who are acknowledged as leaders often are nurtured and guided by others, seek and function in environments that encourage leadership behavior, "test" the role, and study others who have been leaders.

Thus, the development of oneself as a leader is a purposeful process that is enhanced by guidance and support from others, but what are the ways in which one can develop leadership skills? This chapter explores numerous approaches to leadership development, and several of the strategies that have particular relevance for nurses are examined in depth.

GENERAL APPROACHES TO LEADERSHIP DEVELOPMENT

Emergence as a leader is a developmental learning process in which capacities, insights, and skills gained through one experience or at one level serve as the basis for further growth; thus, leaders go through stages in their development. It also is generally acknowledged that one learns to be a leader by serving as a leader. Merely talking about being a leader or observing others in that role does not make one a leader. One is a leader when he or she exercises leadership.

Based on past performance or promise of future performance, one often is expected to provide leadership to a group. As a person has success in that role, more and more leadership is expected of that individual; thus, one may continually be "promoted" to higher levels of leadership responsibility.

Finally, leadership development is a lifelong process. As nurses progress throughout their careers, they will face new challenges. The need for change will always exist, and groups will need leaders to help them weather the forces of change. Conflict also will always exist, particularly as resources become more scarce and new healthcare workers challenge traditional roles; groups will need leaders to help them manage those conflicts. New visions will continually need to be articulated, as previous visions are realized or changing societal expectations demand new directions; groups will need leaders to help them see and realize those new visions. As the circumstances of our lives are constantly altered, our leadership skills also need to be refined, renewed, and further developed.

Lecture and Discussion: Formal Course Work

Perhaps one of the most common and easiest ways to develop leadership skills is through participation in lectures, discussions, or formal course work on leadership. Such experiences provide information about the phenomenon, facilitate a "formal" examination of individuals who have demonstrated leadership in the past or in contemporary society, and stimulate thinking about the nature of leadership and followership. Participation in an effective discussion group also provides experience in working with others to reach decisions and helps one develop an awareness of the need for more than single, simple answers to complex problems.

In addition to individual or clusters of lectures and discussions about leadership, many universities have instituted programs that focus on leadership. The University of Richmond (Virginia) offered the first baccalaureate program in leadership in 1992, and Chapman University (California) and Fort Hays State University (Kansas) have since added their own majors in this field. Kennesaw State University (Georgia) offers a master's degree in conflict management, and Antioch University (Ohio) offers a master's in conflict resolution and a doctoral program in leadership and change in the professions. Duke University's (North Carolina) advertisements note that strong leadership is the best way to ensure success, and they offer an innovative leadership program to prepare individuals for that role. The University of Denver's (Colorado) Pioneer Leadership Program (Reisberg, 1998) combines classroom instruction with adventure-based outings as a way to develop leadership abilities, and it leads to a minor in leadership studies. A growing number of institutions now offer minors in leadership studies, many more than were listed in a source book of courses and programs in leadership (Schwartz, 1998), that was developed to document the growth of such opportunities.

In 1992, the National Student Nurses Association (NSNA) developed an independent study module that was intended to serve as a model for schools to involve students as active participants in learning about leadership, developing leadership skills, and enhancing professional socialization. Through individualized learning contracts with faculty members, students use their experiences as the chairperson of a local Student Nurses Association (SNA) chapter or committee to study their own leadership style, gain confidence when leading groups, appreciate the many facets of group decision-making, and understand the legislative process. This has now evolved to the NSNA Leadership University (*www.nsnaleadershipu.org/nsnalu*).

Finally, many nursing education programs have credit-bearing courses or noncredit workshops that deal with leadership and its development, and many use creative strategies to help those concepts "come alive" for students (Kirkpatrick, Brown, Atkins, & Vance, 2001; Valiga & Bruderle, 1997). Individuals wanting to learn more about this complex concept and the effective exercise of leadership, particularly in nursing and healthcare, may benefit from enrolling in such courses; however, it would be wise to study the course offering carefully before enrolling to be certain that it does indeed focus on leadership rather than on management. In addition, one might benefit from looking at "old" things (e.g., movies such as *12 Angry Men, Gung Ho*, or *One Flew Over the Cuckoo's Nest*) with "new" eyes and new perspectives.

One study (Levine, 2005) examined graduate programs in education to determine their effectiveness in preparing school leaders. Such academic programs have been in existence for many years, and they have produced principals and superintendents who have led our nation's schools and school districts. Despite this success, it was determined that at a time when "the quality of leadership in our schools has seldom mattered more" (p. 5), and in "an era of profound social change" (p. 5), "fundamental rethinking of what [graduate] schools [in education] do and how they do it" (p. 5) was required. Thus, while formal course work in leadership is a viable route to development in this area, one must look carefully at the quality of those learning experiences to ensure they are relevant and effective.

Role-Playing and Simulation

Although it often makes people uncomfortable, participation in role-playing or simulation exercises is an excellent way to develop leadership skills. By being expected to play the role of leader, one must be articulate, forward-thinking, creative, able to manage conflict and resolve differences among group members, acknowledge and build on the strengths of followers, and help the group move forward. Role-playing also can serve as a "diagnostic technique," through which one's strengths and areas needing improvement become apparent. For example, it will be evident if the individual playing the role of leader cannot articulate a vision clearly; the individual will then know that this is a particular skill needing more development.

Role-playing and simulation also can serve as a way to "test" various solutions to problems before actually being in the problem situation. For example, a group might construct a scenario in which one of their members plays the passive "sheep" follower role (Kelley, 1992) and the leader must figure out ways to help that follower become more effective. Knowing that reality often presents leaders with many "sheep" followers, being able to address this situation through role-playing gives leaders an opportunity to generate a number of approaches to dealing with such a situation before finding themselves actually faced with it. In addition, this kind of experience provides other participants with an opportunity for vicarious learning in which they have observed which strategies were successful and which were not.

Sensitivity Training

Participation in sensitivity training sessions led by expert facilitators provides participants with an opportunity to focus on openness, how hostilities and defensiveness may be exhibited within a group, and one's personal feelings, perceptions, and biases. It also increases one's sensitivity to others' needs and helps one appreciate the significance of shared decision-making. Finally, such sessions also assist group members to reflect on the inner workings or processes of the group itself: who assumed what kinds of roles, who emerged as the leader, who was most effective in moving the group forward and why, and so on. Such insights are invaluable for those who will provide leadership in their work settings, professional associations, or communities.

> *There's nothing wrong with a pleasant, good natured approach to people and problems—in fact, there's none better. The strange thing is that we so often forget to use it.* —Dwight Eisenhower

Role Modeling

Effective leadership skills can be developed by carefully observing individuals who are successful as leaders. By studying what such people do, how they communicate, how they motivate followers to "join in the cause," their level of energy and personal investment, their ability to keep the group focused on the vision despite conflicts and challenges along the way, and how their careers have evolved can be extremely helpful to the novice leader.

Role modeling occurs whether or not it is planned or purposeful. In other words, many of us pattern ourselves after others, even though we may not be aware of such unconscious "decisions," and we may find that we have adapted the negative or nonhelpful behaviors exhibited by others, as well as the positive or helpful ones. Therefore, role modeling is much more effective when it is done consciously and with deliberation.

Conscious or "formal" role modeling may be enhanced by attending professional conferences and conventions where one observes how participants conduct themselves, deal with "hot" issues that are open to debate, express opinions, and "connect" with members of the audience. It also can be achieved by being more observant during meetings. Who is typically able to convince the group that his or her point is the one that should be supported, and what does that person do that makes him or her so convincing? Conscious role modeling occurs when one reads articles or editorials written by nurse leaders and reflects on their communication style, their willingness to address controversial topics publicly, and the fact that they use print media to convey a strongly held message or articulate a vision. Finally, leadership can be facilitated by reading biographies about leaders—in nursing (such as the 23 leaders presented by Houser & Player, 2004, 2007) or outside nursing, contemporary or historical—and studying what they did and how they did it.

Institutes and Fellowships

A more formalized approach to leadership development occurs through participation in institutes and fellowships. Such opportunities are announced in professional publications and are open to a wide variety of individuals.

In 1998, for example, the American Academy of Nursing and the American Nurses Foundation formed a partnership to develop an Institute for Nursing Leadership. The aim of this institute was to "build new leadership capacities through self-assessment, skill-building learning modules, and programs designed to connect nurses with mentors, sponsors and other . . . contacts" (Ferguson, 1998, p. 10). It was multi-focused and relevant to nurses at all stages of their careers: fostering leadership skill building among undergraduate and graduate nursing students, fostering leadership competencies for nurses at early and emerging career points, facilitating mentoring and networking for nurses in their first managerial position, brokering access to leadership development programs (with executives outside their traditional work settings) for senior executive nurses, and enhancing connections with leaders in the field to maintain leadership capacity in the profession.

Sigma Theta Tau International, the Honor Society of Nursing, has as one of its major goals the development of leadership among its members. The ultimate purpose of focusing on leadership is to promote the discovery, dissemination, and utilization of knowledge to improve the health of individuals and communities worldwide. Through its workshops, programs, conferences, and International Leadership Institute, Sigma Theta Tau International serves to address the leadership development needs of nurses who are currently providing leadership at the local, regional, and international level as well as nurses who have the potential to provide such leadership. The goal of the Institute is to help nurses "be able to influence people, organizations and situations to bring about transforming change" (*Annual Report 1999*, p. 7).

Florida Atlantic University offers a Nursing Leadership Institute, a community/ university partnership designed to help nurse leaders enhance their leadership skills through continuing education programs and sharing of best practices, as well as a Novice Nursing Leadership Institute, another practice/education partnership designed to create a pool of future nursing leaders. In Boston, a consortium of Harvard-affiliated nursing services created the Institute for Nursing Healthcare Leadership (INHL) to "foster international nursing leadership in developing solutions to the problems created by the intersection of rapidly changing healthcare systems, aging patient populations, and a world-wide nursing workforce shortage" (*www.inhl.org*).

The West Virginia Nursing Leadership Institute is a 12-month program designed to prepare nurses to become effective leaders who can—and will—address and positively affect the critical need for nurse recruitment and retention in their communities and beyond. The Central Virginia Nursing Leadership Institute is an innovative community-wide, year-long experience that builds on management leadership skills in mid-level nurse managers from all sectors of healthcare, and similar programs exist in Kansas and Kentucky for public health nurses, and in North Carolina for school nurses. The University of Illinois at Chicago's International Center for Health Leadership Development conducts leadership development activities that prepare leaders from communities, community health centers, and health professions education to build links and partnerships between communities and institutions. It helps individuals discover their leadership capabilities and helps them see that, in many ways, leadership is a function of the relationship between leaders and followers.

Another program in nursing that focuses on the development of leadership is the Leadership Initiative for Nursing Education (LINE) program, originally funded by the Helene Fuld Health Trust. This initiative includes a 6-month fellowship and a 5-day leadership institute designed to enhance the leadership skills of both nurse educators and nursing students at the baccalaureate level and to promote closer relationships between nurse educators and employers, who seek to hire graduates prepared for the leadership challenges of this century.

Finally, several prestigious leadership programs are sponsored by nonprofit foundations including the Kellogg Leadership for Community Change program, the Pew Partnership for Civic Change, the Ford Foundation's Leadership for a Changing World program, and the Rockefeller Foundation's Next Generation Leadership fellowships (Joslyn, 2002). In addition, the Center for Creative Leadership (North Carolina) is a well-established program that offers workshops, books, and other resources to positively transform the way leaders, their organizations, and their societies confront the most difficult challenges of the 21st century.

All these and many more programs are designed to enhance leadership development. When combined with "on-the-job training" and extensive reflection and self-assessment efforts, individuals can be most effective in developing as leaders in their organizations, communities, and professions.

On-the-Job Training

Perhaps the most effective way to develop as a successful leader is to use such skills "on the job." On-the-job training may include temporary job rotations to positions that require the use of new skills, assignment as an assistant or apprentice to someone in a leadership role, serving as the chair-elect of a committee, or participation in some leadership internship, such as those described previously or those offered through one's employing agency. On-the-job training also may occur through a mentor relationship, a concept discussed in more depth later in this chapter.

Knowing is not enough; we must apply. Willing is not enough; we must do. —Goethe

Reflection and Self-Assessment

Reflection is generally viewed as having two dimensions: "reflecting on experience after an event occurs and reflection in action—in real time—during an event" (Johns, 2004, p. 24). It involves learning from everyday experiences and gaining insights about oneself and one's actions. By thinking deeply and honestly about your vision, your character, your passion, your ability and willingness to share power, the way you communicate, your persistence, the extent to which you embrace and celebrate differences and other qualities of effective, transformational leaders, you can identify the strengths you wish to enhance and the limitations you wish to improve as a leader.

Such insights also occur through serious and thoughtful completion of self-assessment tools and careful reflection on what they reveal about you. The *Self Profile* (1987), for example, can help you identify how you relate to others, how you might respond in a given situation, and how you can build more meaningful relationships with others. *Self Profile* statements such as the following offer insights to leadership behaviors and may be particularly revealing: "When in a group, I tend to speak and act as the representative of that group," "When faced with a leadership position, I tend to actively accept that role rather than diffuse it among others," "It's important to me that people follow the advice that I give them," and "Other people usually think of me as being energetic."

Thus, reflection and self-assessment are important strategies to leadership development and should be integral to the ongoing development of any leader. Seeking feedback from peers and potential followers also is useful in assessing your leadership qualities.

Summary

In essence, nurses who are seeking to develop or enhance their leadership skills and abilities would benefit from attending carefully to those in their work and professional environments (e.g., as potential role models) and considering becoming involved in some type of formal leadership training program. In selecting such a program, one should look for opportunities to examine the complex phenomenon of leadership in depth, be certain one chooses carefully between leadership development and management training programs, and choose a program that provides opportunities to actually experience the role of leader; receive thoughtful, critical feedback on one's performance in that role; and receive guidance in building on areas of strength and developing areas of weakness. Potential and effective nurse leaders also would be best served by practicing in an environment that facilitates their development as leaders. The following case study illustrates how one can purposefully pursue development as a leader, as well as how lack of planning can result in missed opportunities and delayed or limited development in the role.

Case Study in Developing as a Leader: Planned and Unplanned

Marty and Josh were classmates during their nursing program and upon graduation, both went to work at the local medical center. While they both enjoyed successful careers in nursing, each evolved to a very different place in terms of his leadership and the extent of his influence in the field.

Both Marty and Josh identified Dr. Richards as one of the best teachers they had in nursing. She was knowledgeable in the subject she taught but admitted to not knowing things and thought those situations through "out loud," so students could benefit from her thinking processes. She used innovative strategies to facilitate learning and actively engaged students in designing their own learning experiences. Dr. Richards had published extensively in her area of expertise, completed research that influenced patient care, had been inducted into the American Academy of Nursing and received numerous awards, consulted with schools of nursing across the country, was invited to speak at national and international conferences, was actively involved in her specialty organization, and most recently was inducted into the National League for Nursing's Academy of Nursing Education. While she did not brag about these accomplishments, Dr. Richards kept her students informed about her activities and the directions in which her career took her.

While neither Marty nor Josh thought they would pursue an academic position, they were impressed with Dr. Richards' accomplishments and contributions, and they often talked about their desire to have a career that is as exciting and productive as hers. Marty took steps to make that happen. Josh did not.

While still a student, **Marty** took advantage of the opportunity to talk with Dr. Richards (and other faculty) about their careers, how they balanced professional development activities with work responsibilities, and how they got where they are. He asked for advice about jobs, how to get involved in professional organizations, who the "movers and shakers" were in his area of interest (rehabilitation), how to get the most out of conferences one attends, and whether Dr. Richards would mentor him, particularly at the outset of his career. He wrote goals for where he would like to be 5 and 10 years after graduation and began to outline steps to achieve those goals. As an RN, Marty volunteered to serve on several committees at the rehab center where he worked, proposed innovations in patient care that evolved from research reports he read, submitted abstracts for presentation of those patient care innovations at the national convention of the nursing rehabilitation organization, sought feedback from peers and supervisors about his practice, challenged ideas presented by others and offered alternative solutions, and worked with his mentors to advance professionally. Ten years after graduation, Marty was well-known in the field of rehabilitation nursing, was collaborating with experts in that field to design and implement research projects, and was reporting the findings from their research in journal articles and at conferences. Rehabilitation nurses across the country knew of Marty's work and used his research findings and ideas about innovative practices as the basis for their own practice. Without question, Marty was a leader in the field whose own work influenced the work of others and helped shape a preferred future for rehabilitation nursing practice.

Josh, on the other hand, never sought out his teachers while he was a student or afterwards. He was dedicated to providing excellent care to the homeless, but he made no effort to actively shape that practice or advocate for the population he served daily. When asked to attend a meeting about care of the homeless, Josh accepted, listened attentively, and prepared a comprehensive report of what took place during that meeting; however, he made no special effort prior to the meeting to be best prepared for it, did not contribute to the discussion, did not take risks to offer different perspectives (despite the fact that he disagreed with some of what was being proposed), and did not influence the thinking of those at the table. While he knew of several organizations that worked diligently on behalf of the homeless, Josh did not join or actively participate in any events sponsored by those organizations. He also did not attend professional conferences on the topic, attempt to incorporate research findings into his practice, challenge his colleagues to continually strive for excellence, seek out a mentor, nor expand his professional networks. The care he provided was exceptional, but his sphere of influence was extremely limited, and his plan to advance as a leader was essentially nonexistent.

ENVIRONMENTS THAT FACILITATE LEADERSHIP DEVELOPMENT

Aspiring leaders may not be in a position to create an environment that facilitates leadership development. However, they may be in a position to choose to practice and participate in such environments. What do such environments look like? What should nurses look for in such environments?

Much like those that promote creativity (see Chapter 5) and human development in general, environments that promote the development and enhancement of leadership skills and abilities are open, trusting, and dynamic. In such environments, individuals feel free to raise questions about what is being done, how it is being done, why it is being done in a particular way, and why it is being done at all. Not only is a questioning attitude accepted, it is encouraged and expected. Bennis (2004) refers to this as a "culture of candor."

Environments that promote the development of leadership do not maintain the status quo and do not put individuals into "boxes," but they do encourage each person to reach his or her maximum potential. A spirit of competitiveness that constantly pushes members to achieve excellence may characterize the environment, but group members are not in competition with each other. Indeed, environments that facilitate the development of leadership recognize the strengths and talents of each member of the group, find ways to build on those strengths, and expect group members to guide, encourage, and support each other as they continue to grow. They are, in essence, environments in which leaders are allowed to emerge and followers are seen as valuable, contributing members of the team.

Individual members of the group are encouraged and expected to take risks and try new roles, even though they may fail. For example, a relatively new nurse may be asked to head up an ad hoc committee that is charged to look at how the working relationships between licensed and unlicensed personnel can be enhanced. With the guidance and support of the nurse manager or more seasoned nurses on the unit, this new nurse would be expected to take the lead in working with group members to formulate the goals for this group, suggesting ways the group could go about achieving those goals, maintaining open communications with other nurses not directly involved in the project about the progress of the committee, and keeping the group focused on preparing a timely report that includes realistic, feasible recommendations for how working relationships can be enhanced. Along the way, this nurse may make some mistakes, but he or she has been provided with an opportunity to develop leadership skills and to think of himself or herself as a leader.

I view mistakes as opportunities to learn. —Zerrie Campbell

An environment that facilitates leadership development does not "recycle" the same people over and over again, giving only a limited number of individuals an opportunity to grow. Although there is some merit in "recycling" leaders (Kelly, 1991; Stocker, 1991) (e.g., organizations that do this make the best use of people who have proven themselves to be effective, and they benefit from the experience and history of these individuals), repeated recycling with limited opportunities for involvement of inexperienced nurses does not serve the profession well in the long run because it does little to contribute to the ongoing development of leaders.

Finally, a leadership development environment is characterized by good channels of communication and a sense that all members are free to suggest ideas (e.g., they do not merely wait for the person "in charge" to generate ideas). It "forces" members to address issues of significance to them and the profession, and it encourages the sharing of information, rather than the hoarding of it. The Leadership Environment Assessment Survey (Table 9–1) can be used to help analyze the extent to which one's work settings or professional organizations can facilitate the development of leadership.

TABLE 9-1 Leadership Environment Assessment Survey

Think about your place of employment or a professional organization in which you are involved (e.g., your state nurses' association, your clinical specialty group, your local honor society). With that organization in mind, consider each of the following questions about the nature of the general environment or "culture." **Yes** responses to most questions suggest that the organization supports, encourages, and expects leadership among its members. **No** responses to most questions may suggest that the organization's priorities do not include leadership development.

QUESTION	YES	NO
Is this organization open to new ideas and new ways of doing things?	✓	
Do members of the organization feel free to raise questions about what is being done? How things are being done? Why things are being done at all? Why things are done in a particular way?	✓	
Is a questioning attitude accepted, encouraged, and expected in the organization?		✓
Does the organization prevent putting individuals into "boxes"?		✓
Does the organization push members to strive for excellence?	✓	
Is competition among group members healthy and productive?		✓
Are the strengths and talents of individual members recognized?	✓	
Are the strengths and talents of individual members built upon?	✓	
Are group members expected to guide, encourage, and support each other as they continue to grow?	✓	
Are leaders allowed to emerge in the organization?	✓	
Are followers seen as valuable, contributing members of the group?	✓	
Are individual group members encouraged to take risks and try new things?	✓	
Are mistakes accepted as part of the learning process for group members?	✓	
Are different group members given opportunities to develop as leaders?	✓	
Are channels of communication clear and open?		✓
Are group members allowed and encouraged to address issues that are of significance to them and the profession?	✓	
Is information shared?		✓
Are accomplishments of group members acknowledged and rewarded?	✓	

EMPOWERMENT

The environment that encourages, supports, and expects leadership development can be thought of as an empowering environment. Empowerment is a process through which individuals feel strengthened, in control, and in possession of some degree of power. It often is "given" by someone in a position of power or authority (e.g., a nurse manager, the home health agency supervisor), but it also can be "taken" by an individual.

"Instead of exercising power over people, transforming leaders champion and inspire them" (Burns, 2003, p. 26). This is empowerment, where "leaders encourage followers to rise above narrow interests and work together for transcending goals" (p. 26). In fact, as Burns said, transforming leadership is achieved "not by enslaving followers, but by liberating and empowering them" (p. 27).

When someone in a position of power empowers others, it is through the sharing of that power. People are empowered by others when they are invited to participate in making decisions that will affect their lives, their work, and their futures. Rather than having "Big Brother" make all the decisions because "he knows best," those people who will have to live with the consequences of decisions are involved in making them. It is clear that this model has relevance for the administrator–staff nurse relationship, but it also has relevance for the nurse-patient relationship, the teacher–student relationship, the parent–child relationship, and any other relationship in which one person typically has more power than others.

Nurses are empowered in their organizations when they are held accountable. Rather than being in a position in which blame can be placed on someone else or "the system" for less-than-ideal outcomes, empowered nurses know that the quality of care they deliver is their responsibility and that they are accountable for their actions and inactions. By being held accountable, nurses actually have more power in the practice arena.

Nurses are empowered when a shared governance model is in place. In this environment, nurses set their own schedule, formulate goals for their unit or agency, set standards of excellence, participate actively in peer review, and support one another. The structure is more open and interactive than limiting and hierarchical, and the success or failure of the group is the responsibility of all members, not only the nurse manager or supervisor. Such a model requires that nurses are adequately prepared to assume such responsibility and that there is a mix of skills and experiences in the group to implement the model most effectively.

Although we tend to think of empowerment as something someone in power does for those who are more powerless, that is far from the only means to empowerment. Nurses who find themselves in work or professional environments that are not designed to be empowering can still feel strengthened and "in control" by their own actions.

Empowerment or strength comes from a number of sources. Among the most significant of those sources is knowledge! Nurses empower themselves when they are knowledgeable and expert in their area of practice: when they know the structure, dynamics, and culture of the organizations in which they work; and when they know how to use resources effectively. They also empower themselves when they know themselves: their strengths and limitations, their values and biases, and what motivates them!

Empowerment also comes from having a sense of control over one's life! This may take the form of choosing where one will work; the level of excellence toward which one will strive, regardless, perhaps, of the standards held by others in the setting; and the degree to which one will accept being spoken down to, taken advantage of, or criticized unjustly. To some extent, it is related to self-esteem, self-worth, personal pride, and one's sense of identity.

> *The secret of joy in work is contained in one word— excellence. To know how to do something well is to enjoy it. —Pearl Buck*

Participating actively in one's work setting, professional association, or community also gives one a sense of having control over one's life and is empowering. By serving on committees, for example, nurses are in a better position to influence decisions that are made, and they are able to ensure that nursing's voice is heard; this is empowering. Holding office in a professional association or engaging actively in the debate of issues presented at a convention of that association is empowering because it gives nurses an opportunity to shape the future of the organization and, perhaps, the profession. Meeting with local legislators and community leaders about ways to enhance the resources available to children and the elderly in one's community is empowering because it reinforces one's ability to advocate for and help improve the lives of those who cannot speak for themselves.

Thus, empowerment need not occur only when someone in a position of power or authority decides to "give" some of that power away. Each of us can "take" some power by our own actions. Perhaps we need to return to school for an advanced degree, attend a workshop on assertiveness, volunteer to serve on a committee, run for political office, or review and reaffirm our values related to excellence and quality patient care. Perhaps we also can feel more empowered by entering into a relationship with a mentor.

MENTORING

Mentor was a figure in Greek mythology who served as the wise and faithful guardian and tutor of Telemachus during the 10-year absence of his father, Odysseus, who fought in and struggled to return home from the Trojan War. The words "mentor" and "mentoring," therefore, typically refer to an experienced individual who befriends and guides a less experienced individual.

Although the word "mentor" is often abused today—with anyone who shows the slightest interest in a person or offers the slightest amount of assistance being referred to as a "mentor"—a true mentor invests a great deal of time and effort in the advancement and growth of a protégé. Such a relationship is conscious, purposefully designed, and typically extends over a number of years.

What Is a Mentor?

Mentors are close, trusted, experienced counselors or guides. They are accomplished and more experienced individuals, usually, but not always, in the same profession of the neophyte, and they offer neophytes advice, teach them, sponsor them, and guide them through significant points in their careers. As such, they help protégés establish themselves in the profession.

By serving as a mixture of "good parent" and "good friend," mentors provide counsel during times of stress, encouragement during risk-taking endeavors, intellectual challenges, and assistance in the development and enhancement of professional skills. They encourage, cajole, test, teach by example, advise, model, act as a partner, sponsor, and give honest feedback, both positive and negative.

Mentors see some potential in a neophyte, which the neophyte often does not see in herself or himself, and then they do something about that potential. The "something" mentors do is to commit themselves to the neophytes, often for a number of years: helping them develop a clearer professional identity, fostering their growth in personal and professional power, supporting and facilitating the realization of their dreams, and acting as an energizer and a sounding board.

Mentors also inspire neophytes and challenge them to achieve a level of professionalism they may not have known otherwise. By representing a point of development to which neophytes aspire, mentors invite their protégés into a new world, as peers and colleagues, and open doors for them. They help their protégés "learn the ropes" within a broadened community of colleagues so that they can sense the political climate, spot the behind-the-scenes actions, gain insights into the profession, expand their networks, and eventually spread their wings and fly.

Myths About Mentors and Mentoring

Mentoring often is thought of as a panacea for solving the problems of nurses in the healthcare arena or women executives aspiring to climb the corporate ladder. Nurses, however, would be wise to be alert to a number of myths surrounding mentors and mentoring (Sandler, 1993):

- *Myth:* The best way to succeed is to have a mentor. *Reality:* Mentoring is important and can make a significant difference in the career development of many individuals, but it is not necessarily essential for success or survival.
- *Myth:* Mentoring is always beneficial. *Reality:* Although there are numerous benefits to a mentoring relationship, there are some limitations as well, such as the difficulty in sustaining the intensity required of both participants over time, the exclusivity of the relationship (e.g., the mentor invests in a very small number of individuals and is not available to work with a larger number of neophytes), the potential for the protégé to rely primarily or exclusively on the mentor for emotional support and guidance rather than interacting with a broader scope of colleagues, and the fact that the mentor, not the protégé, typically "sets the agenda."
- *Myth:* The mentor should be older than the person being mentored. *Reality:* It is quite possible that the more experienced, accomplished individual in the relationship is younger chronologically.
- *Myth:* A person can have only one mentor at a time. *Reality:* Although it may be difficult to maintain close, intense relationships with several mentors simultaneously, it is not impossible. One mentor may be most

effective in helping a neophyte write grants, another may be the expert clinician who gives guidance with difficult clinical problems, and a third may be the best resource in gaining entry to a professional association.

• *Myth:* If you are seeking a mentor, you have to wait to be asked. *Reality:* It is perfectly acceptable for a neophyte to approach a potential mentor to discuss the possibility of entering into a relationship.

• *Myth:* Men are better mentors for women. *Reality:* Most mentors throughout history probably have been men largely because women were not socialized (until recently) in the direction of such relationships and many women were not in positions of leadership to serve as mentors. No evidence supports the claim that men are better mentors. In fact, with women's tendency to attend to personal issues and not merely work or professional ones, a female mentor may be more effective than a male mentor.

• *Myth:* When a man mentors a woman, the chances are great that it will develop into a sexual encounter. *Reality:* This, of course, is a possibility in any relationship, but when the mentoring relationship is focused on the career development and advancement of the protégé, sexuality need not, and, indeed, should not, enter into it.

• *Myth:* The mentor always knows best. *Reality:* Although it is true that the mentor is the wiser, more experienced member of the pair, it also is important to remember that the protégé is a bright, talented individual with ideas and a great deal of potential. Those talents should not be ignored or exploited in the relationship to benefit or stroke the ego of the mentor. The whole point of a mentoring relationship is to promote the career advancement of the protégé, not to make the protégé dependent on the mentor. Thus, the protégé must play a significant role in the relationship and sometimes is the person who "knows best."

What Mentors Look for in Protégés

Mentors and leaders look for novices who have the potential to move the profession ahead. They then invest the time, energy, and caring to create what they believe will be a future leader in the field. With this kind of investment expected of mentors, it is no wonder that they would choose neophytes who show they are worth investing in and are likely to show some measure of reward for the investment made.

Specifically, mentors often seek protégés who possess certain qualities. Table 9–2 presents characteristics that may serve as a guide to determine whether we are the kind of individual in whom a mentor might invest. In essence, mentors look for protégés who are beginning leaders or have the potential to be leaders. They then work to help those individuals develop the knowledge, skills, and savvy needed to be effective leaders.

Caveats Regarding a Mentor Relationship

When considering entering a mentoring relationship, both individuals should consider the following caveats or "commandments" (Sandler, 1993):

TABLE 9-2 What Mentors Look for in Protégés

Mentors often seek protégés who possess certain qualities. The following characteristics may serve as a guide to determine whether you are the kind of individual in whom a mentor might invest:

- Intelligence
- A self-starter: someone who is internally motivated
- Someone who is looking for new challenges
- Good interpersonal and communication skills: someone who is articulate
- A risk-taker
- A hard worker
- Someone who has and understands ideas and is always open to new ideas and possibilities
- Integrity
- Someone who presents himself or herself professionally: in appearance, through the written word, and so on
- A sense of humor
- Someone who is willing to invest in himself or herself
- A curious mind: someone who asks questions and is not satisfied with the status quo
- Someone who has a vision: for himself or herself and for the profession

- Be careful not to confuse a mentor relationship with a personal, emotional one.
- Many people can be mentors—you need not be at the top of your profession to be of assistance to novices.
- The protégé must take personal responsibility for learning.
- The mentor should not be expected to fulfill every need and meet every demand of the protégé.
- The confidences of the mentor must be respected.
- Expectations of both the mentor and protégé (e.g., time, type of assistance) need to be clarified early on in the relationship.
- Protégés should know if they are asking for too much, or too little, of the mentor.
- The feedback from the mentor to the protégé should take the form of praise and constructive criticism, with specific suggestions for improvement.
- The relationship should be used to open doors for future protégés.
- Mentors and protégés need not come from the same type of educational, ethnic, racial, religious, or any other type of background.
- Recognize that the relationship goes through stages—from dependence, uncertainty, and hesitancy to mutual give-and-take to termination, at which point the protégé is more independent and identifies his or her separateness from the mentor.
- Be careful not to fall into mentoring because "it's the thing to do" or the "in" thing.

Benefits to the Mentor

Although it may sound as if the only person who benefits from a mentor relationship is the protégé, nothing could be farther from the truth. Indeed, mentoring is a mutually supportive, mutually beneficial relationship in which the mentor also gains a great deal.

The strength of mentors comes from their own professional experience, self-worth, and autonomy. They must be capable of motivating neophytes to be creative and possess a good sense of their own creative selves. They also must be careful not to direct or control every facet of their protégé's life, and they must be open and willing to learn from the protégé.

As individuals engage in this evolving relationship, the protégé often pursues more sophisticated lines of investigation, develops skills the mentor may not possess, and establishes new networks. The mentor who is open to and willing to learn from a protégé will grow enormously from the relationship.

It is incredibly rewarding for mentors to see novice clinicians, educators, researchers, administrators, and leaders grow and evolve. In many cases, the accomplishments of the neophytes far surpass those of the mentors, and mentors take great pride in seeing their protégés receive awards, make changes in practice, receive offers of significant positions, be elected to office in professional associations, receive competitive grants, and publish articles or books that influence others.

Thus, mentors benefit greatly from working with protégés. The true mentoring relationship is mutually rewarding and results in growth in both individuals. In addition to the personal growth one experiences, both individuals also expand their networks of professional colleagues and "influentials."

NETWORKING

As noted, a mentoring relationship can help both participants develop contacts and expand their professional networks, networks they may call on throughout their careers for assistance, support of ideas, and guidance. Although some take offense at the idea of "using" people to one's benefit, the whole concept of networking is built on the assumption that who one knows is important and can be helpful.

Networks form for the purpose of providing access to contacts, referrals, information, support, feedback, understanding, and empathy. They also can serve to help nurses maintain a social and professional identity and provide a means of working toward organizational, professional, or societal reform.

Nurses might "tap into" their networks when they are looking for a guest speaker for a program, a consultant, someone to fill a key position in an organization, someone to nominate for appointment to a community board, or an expert in a clinical area. They might also use their networks to gather data about practices in other institutions that can help advance a proposal for a change in their own settings. Thus, networks serve a number of useful purposes, without the sustained, intense investment of a mentor relationship.

As described, mentoring is a special kind of relationship between two individuals that is intense, personalized, long lasting, and has positive outcomes for both participants. Indeed, studies have documented several positive outcomes from engagement in a mentoring relationship.

In a classic study of 1,250 top executives, Roche (1979) found that almost two thirds of those studied had mentors, and most mentoring relationships started when the protégé was in his or her 20s or 30s. Roche found that executives who had mentors moved into successful positions more quickly, earned more money at a younger age, were more likely to follow a personal career plan, were better educated, were more satisfied with their career progress, received greater pleasure from their work, and eventually sponsored protégés themselves.

In a classic study of 71 nurse influentials, Vance (1977) found that 83% of those studied had mentors, and 93% of them were consciously aware of being mentors to others. A follow-up study (Kinsey, 1986) revealed similar findings, namely, that many of those nurses who were thought of as influentials in the profession had, themselves, been mentored by others and had served as mentors to novices.

Does everyone need a mentor to "make it" and "get ahead"? No, but most people do need guides, support systems, sounding boards, and peer "pals" to help during certain times throughout their careers, and this is where one's network can be most effective.

Peer "pals" may help each other manage a particularly difficult community health problem or deal with an arrogant physician. *Guides* know easier ways to do something or have experienced a particular situation and share those insights with others. For example, nurses who are enrolled in a master's program may serve as guides to colleagues who are in the process of deciding whether they should pursue graduate education and, if so, what school to attend and what specialty to pursue. Nurses who have particularly good writing skills may review and critique an abstract before it is submitted in response to a "call" for presentation at a conference or a manuscript before it is submitted to a journal for review. *Sponsors* act on behalf of others, promote them, and advance them, much the same way a mentor does, but in more isolated instances, rather than over a lengthy period of time. For example, a faculty member may nominate a graduate for an award or suggest that graduate as a candidate for office in a professional association. All of these are examples of a patron-type system in which nurses "use" their networks but do not necessarily enter into an extended, intense mentoring relationship.

Networks, then, are most effective to enhance one's development as a leader, and nurses should be cautious not to fall into the trap of believing the myths about networking (Cardillo, 2001) outlined in Table 9-3. Instead, we need to broaden our "web" of professional contacts and "use" those contacts to help us face and manage difficult situations, grow professionally, and develop as leaders.

TABLE 9-3 Myths About Networking

- Networking is just for job seekers.
- Networking was a 90s thing.
- You have to leave home to network.
- The Internet has made face-to-face networking passé.
- Networking occurs only in formal arenas.
- Networking is something only managers and executives do.
- You have to personally know someone in a specialty/company to get in.
- Business cards are only for business owners.
- You have to network only with people in your own geographic area.

Source: From Cardillo, D. (2001). Myths about networking. *Nursing Spectrum (New York/New Jersey edition)*, 13A (15), 13.

CONCLUSION

The development of leadership knowledge and skills throughout one's career requires (1) purposeful, goal-directed action; (2) honest, extensive self-assessment; (3) a willingness to ask for assistance or guidance; and (4) a willingness to accept help or guidance when it is offered. It is enhanced by the development and effective use of professional networks, as well as engagement in mentoring relationships.

Nurses who are in positions of influence must take on the responsibility of grooming other promising nurses. Those seeking to be more influential and become leaders must start early to seek experiences and colleagues—and possibly mentors—who will provide the professional and personal nourishment necessary for success. We must identify the people we know who are in a position to help us, let them know we respect their ability, and seek their support. We also must help them see that they have something to gain by helping, guiding, and possibly mentoring us.

> *Whatever development process you're comfortable with, do it to the maximum.* —*Bonnie Saucier*

Each of us must create a personal plan for leadership development throughout our careers and then take responsibility for implementing that plan and documenting the results of various actions, perhaps through maintaining a professional portfolio. Such a plan may include advancing our formal education or enrolling in courses or workshops that will help us develop a better understanding of the phenomenon of leadership or specific skills, such as assertiveness or public speaking. It may include looking for a work setting or professional association that is empowering or one in which strong role models exist. Our personal plan for leadership development may incorporate seeking a mentor, expanding our professional networks, becoming more involved in the political process, running for office in our specialty organization, submitting a manuscript for publication, or responding to a call for paper presentations at a regional or national conference.

Whatever the specific course of action, we will develop as leaders through a well-thought-out plan, and not through the waving of some magic wand. Taking responsibility is a large part of what leadership is all about, and such responsibility grows out of honest self-assessment about our leadership abilities and potentials, as well as positive, focused action. Taking responsibility for our own development as leaders is an excellent way to achieve our professional goals, realize our visions, and shape a preferred future for our profession.

Leaders also are responsible for developing other leaders. Leadership in nursing is about "ensuring a well-thought-through succession plan where the future of the profession remains the key focus" (Ang & Fong, 2003, p. 28).

CRITICAL THINKING EXERCISES

Read at least three journal editorials, one by Leah Curtin, one by Barbara Stevens Barnum, and one by another editor. To what extent do these individuals express controversial ideas and convey a passion about their topic? Do you see any difference in the uniqueness of perspective, challenging nature of the ideas put forth, or passion expressed by the editors? What can you learn from this comparison about the nature of risk taking that is inherent in a leadership role? If you were given the opportunity to write a controversial editorial for a prominent nursing journal, what would you write about? How would you express your ideas? Who would you ask to review your manuscript before you submitted it?

_____

_____

_____

Complete the _Leadership Environment Assessment Survey_ (Table 9–1). To what extent does "your" organization provide an environment that promotes leadership? What can you do to make "your" environment more conducive to the development of leadership skills?

_____

_____

_____

Review the discussion about what mentors look for in a protégé. How do you "rate" in each of the areas listed? What assets do you think you would bring to a mentoring relationship?

_____

_____

_____

List the qualities you would like to see in your mentor. Whom do you know—in your immediate environment, from your educational program, in your specialty organization, in your local community, through your professional readings—that possesses all or most of those qualities? Consider making a contact with that person to discuss the possibility of establishing a mentoring relationship.

_____

_____

_____

Continued

CRITICAL THINKING EXERCISES —*cont'd*

The next time you attend a professional conference or convention, make it a point to meet at least three new colleagues. Talk to each one about his or her interests, areas of expertise, goals, current position, and so on. You also should be prepared to tell them about your goals, interests, and areas of expertise. Exchange e-mail addresses or obtain a business card from each new colleague; note pertinent information about the individual, along with the date and conference where you met the individual; and file it when you return home. This will help you build your professional network.

_____

_____

_____

Reflect on the "results" of the assessments you completed earlier and any other tools you have found. What areas repeatedly emerge as strengths? How can you use those to develop as a leader throughout your career? In what areas do you need to develop? What will you do to overcome those limitations and enhance your leadership potential?

_____

_____

_____

Write your personal career goals: What position would you like to hold 25 years from now? What types of offices would you like to hold? What awards would you like to have won or honors to have been bestowed on you? What types of books or articles would you like to have published? What would you like to be "known for" in the nursing profession? How influential would you like to be on the local, national, and international level? Think big! Now, for each goal, list the types of actions you will need to take to achieve that goal, and plot a timeline for each action. For example, if you would like to publish an article in the *Journal of Nursing Scholarship,* you may want to take an intensive writing course and carefully read the articles published in that journal in the last 5 years to better understand the nature of what is published and its format. Then take a paper you wrote for school or a difficult, challenging patient case study you presented at rounds and rewrite it to fit the guidelines of that journal, and submit it to a former faculty member or a trusted colleague at work for critique and comment. Talk to other nurses who have published in the *Journal of Nursing Scholarship* or other prestigious journals about their experience "breaking into" the publication arena, and seek a mentor to assist you with writing for publication.

_____

_____

References

Ang, R., & Fong, L. C. (2003). Nursing leadership: The Singapore experience. *Reflections on Nursing, 29*(1), 27–28.

Annual Report 1998. (1999). Indianapolis: Sigma Theta Tau International.

Bennis, W. G. (2004). A leadership discussion with Warren Bennis. Webcast sponsored by the American Society of Association Executives Foundation, April 20, 2004.

Burns, J. M. (2003). *Transforming leadership: A new pursuit of happiness.* New York: Atlantic Monthly Press.

Cardillo, D. (2001). Myths about networking. *Nursing Spectrum (New York/New Jersey edition), 13A*(15), 13.

Ferguson, S. L. (1998). Academy, Foundation launch program to enhance nurses' leadership capacity. *The American Nurse, 30*(4), 10.

Gmelch, W. H. (2000). Leadership succession: How new deans take charge and learn the job. *The Journal of Leadership Studies, 7*(30), 68–87.

Houser, B. P., & Player, K. N. (2004). *Pivotal moments in nursing: Leaders who changed the path of a profession.* Indianapolis: Sigma Theta Tau International.

Houser, B. P., & Player, K. N. (2007). *Pivotal moments in nursing: Leaders who changed the path of a profession. Volume II.* Indianapolis: Sigma Theta Tau International.

Johns, C. (2004). Becoming a transformational leader through reflection. *Reflections on Nursing Leadership, 30*(2), 24–26, 38.

Joslyn, H. (2002). Grooming the best and brightest. *The Chronicle of Philanthropy, 14*(23), 35–39.

Kelley, R. (1992). *The power of followership: How to create leaders people want to follow and followers who lead themselves.* New York: Doubleday Currency.

Kelly, L. S. (1991). The conundrum of recycled leadership (Editorial). *Nursing Outlook, 39*(1), 5.

Kinsey, D. C. (1986). The new nurse influentials. *Nursing Outlook, 34*(5), 238–240.

Kirkpatrick, M. K., Brown, S. T., Atkins, A., & Vance, A. (2001). Using popular culture to teach leadership. *Journal of Nursing Education, 40*(2), 90–92.

Levine, A. (2005). *Educating school leaders.* Washington, DC: The Education Schools Project.

Reisberg, L. (1998). Students gain sense of direction in new field of leadership studies. *Chronicle of Higher Education, 45*(10), A49–A50.

Roche, G. (1979). Much ado about mentors. *Harvard Business Review, 58,* 14ff.

Sandler, B. R. (1993). Women as mentors: Myths and commandments (Opinion). *The Chronicle of Higher Education, 39*(27), B3.

Schwartz, M. K. (Ed.). (1998). *Leadership education: A source book of courses and programs.* Greensboro, NC: Center for Creative Leadership.

Self Profile. (1987). Overland Park, KS: National Press Publications.

Stocker, S. (1991). Unraveling the leadership conundrum (Sounding Board). *Nursing Outlook, 39*(4), 188–189.

Valiga, T. M., & Bruderle, E. (1997). *Using the arts and humanities to teach nursing: A creative approach.* New York: Springer.

Vance, C. N. (1977). *A group profile of contemporary influentials in American nursing.* Unpublished doctoral dissertation, Teachers College, Columbia University, New York.

Bibliography

Bos, S. (1998). Perceived benefits of peer leadership as described by junior baccalaureate nursing students. *Journal of Nursing Education, 37*(4), 189–191.

Breaux, A. L. (2002). *101 answers for new teachers and their mentors: Effective teaching tips for daily classroom use.* Larchmont, NY: Eye on Education, Inc.

Curtin, L. (1993). Empowerment: On eagles' wings (Editorial). *Nursing Management, 24*(6), 7–8.

Daloz, L. A. (1999). Mentor: Guiding the journey of adult learners. San Francisco: Jossey-Bass.

Fields, W. L. (1991). Mentoring in nursing: A historical approach. *Nursing Outlook, 39,* 257–281.

Gibson, C. H. (1991). A concept analysis of empowerment. *Journal of Advanced Nursing, 16,* 354–361.

Glennon, T. K. (1992). Empowering nurses through enlightened leadership. *The Journal of Nurse Empowerment, 2*(1), 41–44.

Gunden, E., & Crissman, S. (1992). Leadership skills for empowerment. *Nursing Administration Quarterly, 16*(3), 6–10.

Hartshorn, J. C., Berbiglia, V. A., & Heye, M. (1997). An honors program: Directing our future leaders. *Journal of Nursing Education, 36*(4), 187–189.

Helmuth, M. (1994). Mock convention: A simulation for teaching leadership. *Journal of Nursing Education, 33*(4), 159–160.

Huang, C. A., & Lynch, J. (1995). *Mentoring: The Tao of giving and receiving wisdom.* New York: HarperCollins.

Johnson, W. B., & Ridley, C. R. (2004). *The elements of mentoring.* Hampshire, England: Palgrave Macmillan.

Kelly, L. S. (2000). Where leaders are born: Living the mentoring continuum. *Reflections on Nursing Leadership, 26*(3), 8–9, 46.

Kessenich, C. R. (1997). The evolution of a leadership course. *Journal of Nursing Education, 36*(6), 301–303.

Klein, E., & Dickenson-Hazard, N. (2000). The spirit of mentoring. *Reflections on Nursing Leadership, 26*(3), 19–22, 46.

Krichbaum, K. (1997). Preparing students for leadership in practice. *Creative Nursing, 2,* 12–14.

McCall, M. W., Jr. (1998). *High flyers: Developing the next generation of leaders*. Boston: Harvard Business School Press.

Murray, M. (2001). *Beyond the myths and magic of mentoring: How to facilitate an effective mentoring process*. San Francisco: Jossey-Bass.

Olson, R. K., & Vance, C. N. (1993). *Mentorship in nursing: A collection of research abstracts with selected bibliographies—1977–1992*. Houston: University of Texas Printing Services.

Prestholdt, C. O. (1990). Modern mentoring: Strategies for developing contemporary nursing leadership. *Nursing Administration Quarterly, 15*(1), 20–27.

Shea, G. F. (1999). *Making the most of being mentored*. Boston: Course Technology, Inc.

Shea, G. F., & Woodbury, D. (2001). *Mentoring*. Cincinnati, OH: Muska & Lipman Publishing.

Sinetar, M. (1998). *The mentor's spirit: Life lessons on leadership and the art of encouragement*. New York: St. Martin's Press.

Stewart, B. M., & Krueger, L. E. (1996). An evolutionary concept analysis of mentoring in nursing. *Journal of Professional Nursing, 12*(5), 311–321.

Stoddard, D.A., & Tamsay, R. (2003). *The heart of mentoring: Ten proven principles for developing people to their fullest potential*. Colorado Springs, CO: NavPress Publishing Group.

Taylor, D. E., Barrick, C. B., & Harrell, F. H. (1994). Preparing students for health care reform: An innovative approach for teaching leadership/management. *Journal of Nursing Education, 33*(5), 230–232.

Tebbitt, B. V. (1993). Demystifying organizational empowerment. *Journal of Nursing Administration, 23*(1), 18–23.

Tenner, E. (2004). The pitfalls of academic mentorships. *The Chronicle of Higher Education, 50*(49), B7–B10.

Tracey, C., & Nicholl, H. (2006). Mentoring and networking. *Nursing Management, 12*(10), 28–32.

Vance, C. (2000). Discovering the riches in mentor connections. *Reflections on Nursing Leadership, 26*(3), 24–25, 46.

Vance, C. (2000). Mentoring at the edge of chaos. *Nursing Spectrum, 12A*(17), 6.

Vance, C. (2001). The value of mentoring. *Imprint, 48*(2), 38–40.

Vance, C., & Olson, R. K. (Eds.). (1998). *The mentor connection in nursing*. New York: Springer.

Wilson, B., & Laschinger, H. K. (1994). Staff nurse perception of job empowerment and organizational commitment. *Journal of Nursing Administration, 24*(4), 39–47.

Yoder, L. (1990). Mentoring: A concept analysis. *Nursing Administration Quarterly, 15*(1), 9–19.

Zachary, L. J., & Daloz, L. A. (2000). *Mentor's guide: Facilitating effective learning relationships*. New York: John Wiley & Sons.

Zachary, L. J., & Koestenbaum, P. (2005). *Creating a mentoring culture: The organization's guide*. San Fransicso: Jossey-Bass.

CHAPTER 10

Conclusion

LEARNING OBJECTIVES
- Analyze the concept of excellence.
- Discuss the responsibility for promoting excellence that rests with leaders who will create nursing's preferred future.
- Examine the interrelationship among leadership, excellence, and professional involvement.
- Propose strategies for exercising leadership, promoting excellence, and being professionally involved to create nursing's preferred future.

INTRODUCTION

One of the responsibilities of those leaders who will create nursing's preferred future is to promote excellence. As nursing professionals, we certainly have a responsibility to strive for excellence in our own practice and in the delivery of healthcare to consumers. As leaders who will create a future for nursing that acknowledges and takes full advantage of the myriad talents nurses bring to the healthcare arena, we have an even greater responsibility to promote excellence.

This chapter examines the concept of excellence in depth. Excellence is then related to leadership, and the role of leaders in advancing the notion of excellence is explored. Finally, both concepts—excellence and leadership—are blended with the idea of professional involvement throughout one's career as a means to promote nursing and create a preferred future for our profession.

The two case studies presented depict two very different approaches to an individual's nursing career—one that accepts mediocrity and makes no attempt to be a leader and the other that is characterized by excellence and leadership. Referring back to these case studies as the concept of excellence is discussed and as it is related to

---

Case Studies

ADRIENNE'S CAREER TRACK WHEN SHE IS WILLING TO ACCEPT MEDIOCRITY AND THE STATUS QUO

Adrienne completed a baccalaureate program in nursing 8 years ago. In that time, she has worked in her local community hospital and now holds the position of nurse manager of a 30-bed telemetry unit in the area medical center. She runs her unit very efficiently, patient care is good with few incident reports being filed, and when she attends the mandatory management team meetings of the nursing department, Adrienne reads all material in advance and listens attentively. She occasionally reads a few articles in journals that colleagues bring to the unit, attends all required in-service sessions, and implements new practices as directed by her supervisor. Adrienne does not, however, attend conferences or workshops to advance her learning, is not enrolled in a graduate program, has never sought out a mentor, does not propose new ideas to her staff or at the management team meetings, does not hold membership in her professional association, and is glad to go home at the end of the day, knowing that everything is in order and she does not need to think about her practice until tomorrow.

ADRIENNE'S CAREER TRACK WHEN SHE STRIVES FOR EXCELLENCE AND IS A LEADER

Adrienne completed a baccalaureate program in nursing 8 years ago. In that time, she has worked in her local community hospital and now holds the position of nurse manager of a 30-bed telemetry unit in the area medical center. She runs her unit very efficiently, patient care is good with few incident reports being filed, and when she attends the mandatory management team meetings of the nursing department, Adrienne reads all material in advance and listens attentively. She also, however, always goes to those meetings having read about the latest research in her area of nursing practice and having talked with her staff about ways to improve patient care. She shares those ideas, as well as proposals for how change can be implemented in the institution. Adrienne sought out her former nurse manager as a mentor, and she regularly communicates with her mentor about nursing practice issues, career advancement, and other professional matters. In addition, she serves as a mentor to a former colleague who is beginning her career in nursing. Adrienne seeks out opportunities to attend conferences and workshops as a way to learn more and expand her professional networks, and she participates actively in her professional organization at the state level. She aspires to become involved at the national level and is talking with her mentor and others in the organization about how to make that happen. Adrienne is enrolled in a graduate program in nursing administration and has talked with the chief nursing officer about becoming involved in some system-wide change projects that will be implemented at the institution, offering to read and compile background information that will be helpful to the project team. She looks forward to the day when she can be more actively involved in interdisciplinary research studies related to excellence in nursing care delivery to patients with chronic illness and their families.

leadership and professional involvement should help those ideas come alive for the reader.

> *The rewards of excellence do not come easily; it requires rigorous discipline to achieve them.* —*Edgar Dale*

THE CONCEPT OF EXCELLENCE

"Excellence" is a word we hear tossed about everywhere recently. General Motors says they are in the business of excellence. IBM claims they are all about excellence. The American Nurses Association (ANA) talks about excellence in clinical practice. The National League for Nursing (NLN) promotes excellence in nursing education. Sigma Theta Tau International advances excellence in scholarship. Our colleges and universities talk about excellence in their program offerings, faculty, students, and facilities. What is excellence? What is meant by this often-used, but little-examined, word?

Excellence means striving to be the very best you can be in everything you do—not because some teacher or parent or other "authority" figure pushes you to do that but because you cannot imagine functioning in any other way. It means setting high standards for yourself and the groups in which you are involved, holding yourself to those standards despite challenges or pressures to reduce or lower them, and not being satisfied with anything less than the very best.

This kind of perspective or approach applies to all spheres of life—writing papers for a course, preparing for a final examination, providing care to elderly patients in a long-term care facility, teaching school-age children about good nutrition or sexually transmitted diseases, driving a car, or working to secure more resources for the homeless in our community. Individuals who are committed to excellence do not—and will not—settle for second best, mediocre performance, or "getting by."

> *In all that you do, reflect the excellence that's in you.*
> —*Martin Luther King Jr.*

When we allow ourselves and the systems in which we function to simply be "OK," "good enough" or minimally adequate, we sell ourselves short, and we do little to advance the profession of nursing and ensure quality of care for patients, families, and communities. We fail to be challenged; we fail to grow; we fail to make change; and we fail to help others develop. Excellence means not allowing this state of affairs to exist!

Excellence also means being unwilling to accept the status quo. Wergin (2003, p. xiii) argued "the most useful way to build and sustain a culture of excellence is to create a culture of critical reflection and continuous improvement." Critical reflection, however, does not mean that all one does is criticize the way things are being done and then walk away in the hopes that someone else will correct what is wrong. Instead, individuals who strive for and expect excellence question and challenge the status quo by asking why things are done the way they are, examining the assumptions that underlie existing practices, and offering thoughtful and realistic alternatives for how things could be done in other ways. They are also willing to invest time and energy to implement those alternatives, evaluate their effectiveness, and orchestrate change so that those new approaches become integral to the system.

> *Look for the ideal, but put it into the actual.*
> —*Florence Nightingale*

Excellence means to excel—to surpass—to be the best. It can be equated with accuracy, flawlessness, and even perfection—terms with which many of us are uncomfortable. Indeed, for many, perfection and the pursuit of excellence represents the "impossible dream." But in a piece about perfection in organizations, Mescon and Mescon (1984) noted that "the pursuit of perfection is a challenge and a chase that must be won . . . . We must put to rest the notion that excellence represents fantasy, not fact in organizational life today" (p. 94). Perhaps this statement could be modified to say that "we must put to rest the notion that excellence represents fantasy, not fact in nursing practice today!" According to these authors, "nothing but perfection is acceptable, [and] nothing but perfection should be rewarded" (p. 94).

> *The real voyage of discovery consists not in seeking new landscapes, but in having new eyes.* —Marcel Proust

Excellence is not an "impossible dream." In fact, if we look at just what excellence is, we see it is not so foreign or so unattainable. Many people have written about excellence, but the description of that concept offered by Diers and Evans (1980) many years ago **still** is particularly helpful. These authors said that excellence involves several things:

- *Discipline:* drawing on our knowledge and experience to practice in a "systematic" way that is of the highest caliber; in other words, "not settling for second best"
- *Choreography:* successfully balancing competing demands in our pursuit of goals
- *Responsibility:* acknowledging what we have done well or poorly and blaming no one
- *Caring:* consistently demonstrating a concern and a compassion for others (including our colleagues) and for ourselves
- *Skepticism:* keeping a proper distance from what is thought to be the truth and not accepting everything blindly; keeping our minds open to new ideas, new information, and new approaches
- *Perseverance:* continually striving to fulfill a goal or realize a vision
- *Passion:* "the essence of excellence"; being "inflamed" by our work

> *Let me tell you the secret that has led me to my goal. My strength lies solely in my tenacity.* —Louis Pasteur

Diers and Evans (1980) said "excellent nurses are inflamed by nursing . . . To be an excellent nurse is to be suffused with a deep and almost inexpressible passion for humankind" (p. 30).

Quality is never an accident. It is always the result of high intention, sincere effort, intelligent direction, and skillful execution. It represents the wise choice from among many alternatives.

A commitment to pursuing excellence does not just happen; it does not just randomly occur. Doing whatever it is that must be done requires an ongoing attention that is initiated and maintained by top management in an organization.

Management also recruits and may even reward individuals who are committed to excellence and who consistently produce excellent work. Achieving excellence occurs only with individual investment. Top management and "the organization" can do only so much. What each of us needs to remember is that every job is a self-portrait of the person who did it. Each of us, therefore, needs to autograph **our** work with excellence.

> *Excellence is the gradual result of always striving to do better.* —Pat Riley

The pursuit of excellence must be vigorously and relentlessly incorporated into everything we think, say, and do. As Mescon and Mescon (1984) wrote, "it is the little things that count on the road to perfection. But too often it is the little things that we all too often simply forget" (p. 94). The individual who autographs his or her work with excellence does not ignore or forget the little things, just as he or she does not forget the big ones.

Vince Lombardi, former coach of the Green Bay Packers football team, once said, "The quality of a person's life is in direct proportion to his or her commitment to excellence, regardless of the chosen field of endeavor." This is a profound concept when one considers the significant role it suggests excellence plays in our lives.

According to John Gardner (1961), one of the leading experts on leadership, "We must learn to honor excellence (indeed to demand it) in every socially accepted human activity, however humble the activity, and to scorn shoddiness, however exalted the activity. An excellent plumber is infinitely more admirable than an incompetent philosopher. The society which scorns excellence in plumbing because plumbing is a humble activity and tolerates shoddiness in philosophy because it is an exalted activity will have neither good plumbing nor good philosophy. Neither its pipes not its theories will hold water" (p. 102).

> *If a man is called to be a streetsweeper, he should sweep streets even as Michelangelo painted or Beethoven composed music, or Shakespeare wrote poetry. He should sweep streets so well that all the hosts of heaven and earth will pause to say, here lived a great streetsweeper who did his job well.*
> —Martin Luther King Jr.

Each of us who hopes to make a significant contribution to our organization, our profession, our community, or the world needs to make this commitment. The quality of our lives will be enhanced as a result. As Aristotle said, we are what we repeatedly do. Excellence, then, is not an isolated act, but a habit.

As mentioned earlier, excellence needs to be a way of life, and for those who do make it a habit, it sets up a "vicious cycle." In other words, excellence begets excellence—for ourselves and for those around us.

Striving for excellence is highly contagious because peer pressure and collegial influence have powerful effects and because they can usually do more than management ever could. Evidence exists to support this claim. Curtain (1990) reported on studies that showed that nurses who practice on units where excellent nursing is the norm soon are striving and growing to reach the level of excellence demonstrated by their peers. When nurses practice, however, on a unit where the standard of care is poor and everyone is satisfied merely with maintaining the status quo and "getting by," their practice tends to descend to the lowest common denominator on that unit. Thus, the level of excellence found in practice is a function of the collegiality among nurses and the kind of "habits" they have. It is a reflection of the way they challenge and support each other, and the way they practice, repeatedly.

> *I never had a policy: I have just tried to do my best each and every day.* —Abraham Lincoln

Perhaps each of us needs to take what has been referred to as "the mirror test." Look at ourselves in a mirror and ask if we can honestly tell the person we see there that we have done our very best.

Excellence comes from within, and perfection is impossible without that personal investment. If staff tolerate mediocrity in what they do, practice will be mediocre. Management can create an environment that expects, fosters, and rewards excellence, but it is only when each individual in the organization can "pass the mirror test" and honestly say that he or she has done his or her very best that excellence will occur.

Unless we try to do something beyond what we have already mastered, we will never grow. Excellence, therefore, involves challenging ourselves—accepting challenges that are offered to us (e.g., writing a grant proposal, pursuing advancement through your agency's clinical levels, facilitating a research project on your unit, accepting an invitation to speak at a professional meeting or to the media). Excellence also involves seeking new experiences (e.g., asking to serve on a committee, agreeing to have your name placed on a ballot for election to a committee or office, assuming new responsibilities with cross-training, submitting an abstract in response to a call for papers). Excellence is not allowing ourselves to get too comfortable or too complacent or so wrapped up in our "little corner of the world" that we lose this broader perspective.

> *The secret to leadership is . . . bearing the larger picture always in mind. Ask yourself, 'What are we really trying to accomplish?'* —J. Donald Walters

No one ever attains very eminent success by simply doing what is required of her or him. It is the amount and excellence of what is done over and above the required that determines the greatness of ultimate distinction.

In our society and in nursing, we have, for too long, accepted the mundane, promoted the average, and rewarded the mediocre. But the organization or the profession that is going to make a difference—to the recipients of its services and to those providing the service—is the one that prizes the absolute best at all levels. It is the organization that never forgets the ideal of excellence and never loses the aspiration to go beyond the merely "acceptable."

This goal of organizational excellence has been advanced in several projects recently. The Institute for Healthcare Improvement (IHI) offers a program entitled, "Pursuing Perfection: Raising the Bar for Health Care Performance" (IHI, 2007). This program seeks to "dramatically improve patient outcomes in thirteen health systems in the United States and Europe by pursuing perfection in all major care processes," and institutions that wish to pursue perfection may apply to participate in it.

In 2003, Wergin published a book focusing on excellence in academic departments in colleges and universities. He offered data from a number of studies to support his recommendations that, in order to "build and sustain cultures of excellence" (the book's subtitle), academic departments must have a clear direction, fully engage students and faculty, discuss explicit and tacit values, engage in "'difficult conversations' about matters of importance" (p. 128, citing Lucas, 2000), encourage experimentation and reflection, engage in peer collaboration and thoughtful peer review, respect and benefit from differences, and make a commitment to excellence.

Finally, a major work about how higher education can and should take greater responsibility for creating social change (*Leadership reconsidered*, 2000) offered valuable suggestions on the relevance of transformative leadership in higher education, the role of students in providing leadership, and the significance of a quest for excellence. The authors of this report concluded that "we have the power and the opportunity to transform our institutions" (p. 87), but they acknowledged that "perhaps our most limiting beliefs are concerned with what is *possible*" (p. 88) [emphasis in the original]. Thus, each individual needs to take responsibility for providing leadership that will help us achieve excellence in our lives, our institutions, and our society.

It has been said that only those who dare to fail greatly can ever achieve greatly. In other words, it is only when we strive for excellence, for flawlessness, and for perfection that we will achieve it. In that process we may fail; therefore, taking risks is a critical component of achieving excellence. Although we may fail along the way, we need to try because excellence also involves action or execution (Bossidy & Charan, 2002). One anonymous writer put this idea into words by saying that "Some people dream of worthy accomplishments while others stay awake and actually do them."

Having a dream is critical, but it is not enough. Each of us needs to be able to articulate that dream clearly, express it to others, and entice others to work with us to make it become reality. This is the essence of leadership.

LEADERSHIP AND EXCELLENCE

Just as excellence is a complex phenomenon, so too is leadership. As noted earlier, Burns (1978, p. 2), in a classic work on the topic, asserted, "leadership is one of the most observed and least understood phenomena on earth." This assertion was reiterated by Richardson (2000) who noted that "leadership has often escaped precise definition, yet we respect its power to transform and are quickly able to sense its absence" (p. v). Despite a lack of full understanding, however, many elements of leadership are universal, elements that bear reviewing.

First, there is agreement that, unlike management, *leadership is not necessarily tied to a position of authority in an organization.* In other words, there is a need for and opportunities to function as a leader at every level of every organization, society, and institution. One can be a leader as a staff nurse or as a student, just as well as if one is a nurse manager, the vice president for nursing, a faculty member, a dean, or the president of a professional association. In fact, it may be easier to be a leader if one is not in a position of authority because then that individual is not expected to promote any "party line," and it may be easier for him or her to "rock the boat" by raising difficult questions, articulating a vision, and working toward changing the system.

Second, *leadership is a relationship of influence* more than a relationship of authority. People follow leaders by choice, not because they are required to do so.

Perhaps one of the most important characteristics of leaders is that *leaders have a vision;* they see new possibilities, new horizons, and different options. They have some notion of things being able to be better than they are now, regardless of how good they are now. In addition, this vision is their cause or purpose in life, and they are willing to invest enormous amounts of energy to see it realized. Think again about Martin Luther King, Jr., who worked all his life for racial equality and the peaceful resolution of differences. Mother Teresa devoted her life to helping the poor and disenfranchised. Candy Lightner lost her daughter to a drunk driver and established Mothers Against Drunk Driving (MADD); and many other individuals have had a vision of a better world and worked to see it materialize. This is the stuff of which leaders are made. Each of us needs to ask if we are leaders—if we have a vision of a better world.

> *In the quiet hours when we are alone and there is nobody to tell us what fine fellows we are, we come sometimes upon a moment in which we wonder, not how much money we are earning, nor how famous we have become, but what good we are doing. —A.A. Milne*

In accord with this drive toward realizing a vision, *leaders are change agents.* They are innovators who continually challenge the status quo, stick their heads above the crowd and take the risk of being shot down. They strive to keep people and organizations moving forward. Again, each of us needs to ask ourselves if we are leaders—if we work toward positive change.

If leaders are going to be agents of change, they also must be *comfortable with conflict*. In fact, leaders must be able and willing to seek conflict, introduce it if necessary, and use it to achieve the goals of the group. They do not always want to minimize conflict or "sweep it under the rug" because they know that conflict is healthy and it promotes growth in individuals and organizations. Ask yourself if you are a leader—if you can manage the conflict we face in our daily lives and our professional lives.

Leaders are *willing to use intuition* in making decisions, they are *comfortable with ambiguity and uncertainty,* and they are *creative.* They want to see new forms take shape, and they do not need to rely on predictability or rationality. They *see the "big picture,"* are *"telescopic,"* seem to *have a "get-it-all-together" perspective,* and *want to collaborate* with others to achieve goals, rather than having a narrow, limited, self-centered interest or focus. Each of us needs to ask ourselves if we are leaders, if we are creative, if we can tolerate uncertainty, and if we can look beyond our own needs.

Finally, leaders are *characterized by excellence,* and they work to promote excellence in themselves and others. Driven by their vision, they strive to be the best they can be, and they inspire others to do the same. Dissatisfied with the status quo, they take risks, try innovative approaches, call on their creativity, and work to make change. Energized by a desire to continue to grow and learn, they seek new opportunities, take on challenges, and know how to manage conflict. Appreciative of the diverse and complex world in which we live, they do not allow themselves to become too highly specialized or too narrowly focused. "Social change results only when people take it on themselves to get involved and make a difference" (Richardson, 2000, p. iv).

Leaders promote and create excellence, and since "leadership is an essential ingredient of positive social change" (Richardson, 2000, p. iv), leaders create the future.

Ilona Herlinger (1990, p. 4), former president of the interdisciplinary honor society of Phi Kappa Phi, challenged members of that organization to think about what role they would play during the 21st century. The questions she posed are challenges leaders must accept:

- Will you make a significant contribution to or an important difference in the world?
- Will you be a doer or merely an observer?
- Will you be an actor or merely a member of the audience?

In essence, Herlinger challenged us to ponder whether we will strive for excellence or accept mediocrity. She also suggested that we consider whether we will be leaders or apathetic, passive crowd-followers. These ideas are expressed powerfully by Hesselbein (2002, p. 5) who says, "Leadership is a matter of how to *be*, not how to *do* it" (emphasis in original).

PROFESSIONAL INVOLVEMENT

When one thinks about the history of Sigma Theta Tau International, the Honor Society of Nursing, and about the interdisciplinary Honor Society of Phi Kappa Phi, one is inspired by what could be characterized as true leadership and true excellence.

Sigma Theta Tau was started in 1922 by six nursing students who wanted to create some way to recognize and acknowledge nursing scholarship. Phi Kappa Phi was started in 1897 by one young man who dreamed of scholars from all disciplines being recognized on college campuses to the same extent that athletes were recognized. Those six nursing students and that one young man each had a vision, they banded together or enlisted the support of others, they took action and worked tirelessly, and they formed two of the most prestigious honor societies in our country.

Today, each of these organizations has hundreds of chapters and thousands of members. They are dedicated to scholarship and leadership (in the case of Sigma Theta Tau) and to promoting academic excellence (in the case of Phi Kappa Phi). They are proactive and forward-looking. Sigma Theta Tau is international in scope and purpose. Each organization is clear about its purpose; each is focused in its efforts; and each is highly regarded, well respected, and emulated. All of this from a handful of students who saw a need, had a vision, believed in excellence, and exercised leadership.

Members of Sigma Theta Tau are among the most powerful "movers and shakers" in our field. Dorothy Brooten's research on the effects of nursing care on low-birth-weight infants who have been discharged early from the neonatal intensive care unit to home has received accolades from the nursing and medical professions. Lois Evans and Neville Strumpf's extensive work on restraint-free care of the elderly has humanized that care in countless ways. Imogene King's contributions in theory development have been significant in advancing the science of nursing. Melanie Dreher's commitment to advancing the concept of clinical scholarship has been influential in helping nurses in practice develop more significant insights to their practice and be creative in where and how they deliver quality care. Dan Pesut's writings about the future have opened the minds of many. The late Virginia Henderson helped us crystallize the professional nursing role in a way few others have.

> *Real leaders are ordinary people with extraordinary determination.* —Anonymous

By being involved in organizations like this—or in many other professional organizations—each of us has the opportunity to interact with and learn from outstanding individuals. We have the opportunity to see true leaders "in action," connect with and seek possible mentors, be involved in activities that promote excellence, and learn more about ourselves as potential leaders. Individuals such as these have an intense passion for the profession and their own area of work, and they do not hesitate to reach out to, guide, and help others in the field. They share a commitment to advancing the profession in whatever way they can, and they want to invest in others.

Professional involvement also means participating in organizational, community, and political activities to advance our vision and see it become a reality. Nurses who serve on committees where they work, on the board of the local community health center, on school boards, as local freeholders or mayors, or as United States senators, all are in positions of influence and have many opportunities to promote excellence, exercise leadership, and create a preferred future for nursing.

Nurses who publish or give presentations in which controversial ideas are presented or where a high standard of practice is put forth are helping to create nursing's preferred future. The same is true for nurses who conduct special projects (funded or not), conduct research and disseminate the findings, mentor others, and engage in collaborative practice with other nurses and with members of other health-care disciplines. The opportunities to promote excellence and function as a leader are limitless, and each time a nurse engages in activities that advance nursing or that demonstrate leadership to realize a vision, he or she is contributing to the creation of a preferred future for our profession.

CONCLUSION

As we develop as leaders, each of us should take advantage of the opportunities presented to become involved professionally. We might even create opportunities to become involved. Each of us has a responsibility to participate and to try to make a difference. Through networking, role modeling, mentoring relationships, and the continued study of leadership and excellence, practice will be enhanced and we will grow enormously. The outcomes will be excellence in our spheres of practice and a preferred future for the nursing profession that we helped create. Indeed, "leadership holds the key to transforming our institutions . . . and our society" (Richardson, 2000, p. v).

> *When we do the best we can, we never know what miracle is wrought in our life, or in the life of another. —Helen Keller*

In conclusion, a contemporary piece of advice seems to capture the essence of leadership, excellence, and professional involvement:

Excellence can be attained if you . . .

CARE more than others think is wise,
RISK more than others think is safe,
DREAM more than others think is practical, and
EXPECT more than others think is possible.

We hope each student and staff nurse who reads this book will take on the challenges of excellence and leadership. You are the future of our marvelous profession. We have every confidence that you will take up this challenge with all seriousness and that you will succeed in creating a preferred future for nursing.

CRITICAL THINKING EXERCISES

Ask several children how they define excellence or what goes into something being called "excellent." Pose this same question to nurses in practice and to individuals engaged in other professional roles (e.g., teacher, physician, social worker). What common themes emerge in the responses you receive? Are there any differences in the way various groups (e.g., children versus adults, women versus men, nurses versus other professionals) talk about the concept? What conclusions can you draw about why the commonalities and differences exist?

_____

_____

Read a short story or poem or watch a film that has recently received a significant award for excellence, and do the same for a "non-winner" in the genre. What sets the "winner" apart from the "non-winner"? What were or seem to be the criteria used to determine excellence in the area? How do those criteria compare to your personal description/ definition of excellence?

_____

_____

Identify a nurse who recently received an award that acknowledges excellence—in clinical practice, in education, in research, in contributions to the profession, in the care of a particular population (e.g., the homeless), and so on. The award can be local, regional, national, or international. Interview the award recipient about his or her recognition. Talk about the individual's background, philosophy, accomplishments, contributions, and ideas about excellence and leadership. What have you learned from this interview that you can use to promote excellence and exert leadership in your arena of practice? Outline specific strategies that could lead you to receive such an award in the future.

_____

_____

References

Bossidy, L., & Charan, R. (2002). *Execution: The discipline of getting things done.* New York: Crown Publishing Group (Random House).

Burns, J. M. (1978). *Leadership.* New York: Harper Torchbooks.

Curtin, L. (1990). The excellence within (Editorial Opinion). *Nursing Management, 21,* 7.

Diers, D., & Evans, D. L. (1980). Excellence in nursing (Editorial). *Image, 12*(2), 27–30.

Gardner, J. (1961). *Excellence.* New York: Harper & Row.

Herlinger, I. (1990). President's corner. *Phi Kappa Phi Newsletter, 16,* 4.

IHI (Institute for Healthcare Improvement). Pursuing perfection. Accessed October 15, 2007, from *http://www.ihi.org/IHI/Programs/StrategicInitiatives/PursuingPerfection.htm*

Leadership reconsidered: Engaging higher education in social change. (2000). Battle Creek, MI: W.K. Kellogg Foundation.

Mescon, M. H., & Mescon, T. S. (1984). Perfection: The possible dream. *Sky* (Delta Airlines magazine), *13*(9), 94, 96.

Richardson, W. C. (2000). Foreword. In *Leadership reconsidered: Engaging higher education in social change* (pp. iv–vi). Battle Creek, MI: W. K. Kellogg Foundation.

Wergin, J. F. (2003). *Departments that work: Building and sustaining cultures of excellence in academic programs.* Boston: Anker.

APPENDIX

Annotated Bibliography

Adams, R. (1972). *Watership Down*. New York: Avon Books.

Watership Down is a book about rabbits, and the adventures of a group of rabbits who leave their comfortable warren in search of a better, safer place to live. Originally thought of as a children's story, this book is an excellent portrayal of leadership styles, leader/follower interactions, and the qualities of effective leaders and followers.

The group of rabbits that serves as the focal point of the story travels extensively to create a new life for themselves, and they encounter several different warrens along the way. They experience warrens that are leaderless, those that are headed by a totalitarian despot, and those where the "leader" provides direction and the basic needs of rabbits in the warren are met, but there is an aloofness between the leader and followers, and high order needs are not met.

The Watership Down warren rabbits come to form a democratic, participating group where the talents of each rabbit are known and called upon as needed, where followers assume the role of leader when circumstances require a particular type of leadership, and where there is a constant exchange of ideas and support. In essence, this group of rabbits exhibits all that is good about leaders and followers.

This book exposes the reader to various types of leadership and leader-follower relationships. One sees risk-taking, acting in uncertainty, clarity of vision, clear communication, and many other behaviors of leaders . . . all within the context of a beautiful story that captures the imagination and holds one's attention.

Babcock, L., & Laschever, S. (2003). *Women don't ask: Negotiation and the gender divide.* Princeton: Princeton University Press.

When Linda Babcock asked why so many male graduate students were teaching their own courses and most female students were assigned as assistants, her dean said: "More men ask. The women just don't ask." It turns out that whether they want higher salaries or more help at home, women often find it hard to ask. Sometimes they don't know that change is possible — they don't know that they can ask. Sometimes they fear that asking may damage a relationship, and sometimes they don't ask because they've learned that society can react badly to women asserting their own needs and desires.

By looking at the barriers holding women back and the social forces constraining them, *Women Don't Ask* shows women how to reframe their interactions and more accurately evaluate their opportunities. It teaches them how to ask for what they want in ways that feel comfortable and possible, taking into account the impact of asking on their relationships. And it teaches all of us how to recognize the ways in which our institutions, child-rearing practices, and unspoken assumptions perpetuate inequalities . . . inequalities that are not only fundamentally unfair but also inefficient and economically unsound.

With women's progress toward full economic and social equality stalled, women's lives becoming increasingly complex, and the structures of businesses changing, the ability to negotiate is no longer a luxury but a necessity. Drawing on research in psychology, sociology, economics, and organizational behavior as well as dozens of interviews with men and women from all walks of life, *Women Don't Ask* is the first book to identify the dramatic difference between men and women in their propensity to negotiate for what they want. It tells women how to ask, and why they should.

Bass, B. M. (1990). *Bass and Stodgill's handbook of leadership: Theory, research, and management applications* (3rd ed.). New York: The Free Press.

This is a classic volume that provides an historical perspective on leadership, an analysis of the meaning of leadership, descriptions of various categories or typologies of leadership, and an examination of leadership theories and models (including Great Man, trait, situational, psychoanalytic, and other theories). Beyond this introductory material, the major emphasis in this 1000+-page book is on research that has been completed about leaders and leadership.

The research reported focuses on leadership traits, tasks of leaders, leadership styles, women and leadership, leader/follower interactions, and the significance of values to leaders. Concepts such as charisma, inspirational leadership, power, and conflict also are addressed.

This *Handbook* is an excellent resource for any serious student of leadership. Sadly, the book has not been updated since 1990, so current research about leadership is noticeably absent. In addition, although the author notes that leadership and management are different phenomena, most of the studies reported use managers as subjects, thereby suggesting that one needs to be in a position of authority to be considered a leader. Despite these limitations, *Bass and Stodgill's Handbook of Leadership* is a classic that should be read and used as a reference source.

Bass, B. (1985). *Leadership and performance beyond expectations*. New York: The Free Press, MacMillan, Inc.

This outstanding book describes leadership in terms of transformational and transactional components. The author says transformational leadership is found in varying amounts in everyone and needs to be tapped. He offers traditional leaders—such as Moses, Buddha, Jesus Christ, and Mohammed—as well as contemporary leaders—such as Theodore Roosevelt, John F. Kennedy, and Gandhi—as examples for study. He also cites how each of these individuals depicted charisma, individualized consideration, and intellectual stimulation. Bass also gives behavioral examples of transactional leadership and defines the principles of management-by-exception and contingent rewards.

Perhaps the most interesting aspect of this book is the description of the data collected from the author's classic study of 104 military officers who completed the author-developed *Leadership Questionnaire*. This instrument asked the officers about their perceptions of their immediate supervisor's leadership skills, and the findings of what these individuals believed make someone an effective leader is extremely interesting. The results of this study also point out how an effective leader can influence the followers in a group. (A copy of the *Leadership Questionnaire* and parameters for scoring are included in the book.)

Beatty, J. (1998). *The world according to Peter Drucker*. New York: The Free Press.

This book chronicles the life of Peter Drucker and delineates how he constantly pushed himself to become a stronger and more successful person by thinking about what people **can** do, not only what they **cannot** do. Drucker is a firm believer of frequent self-evaluation, which he termed "keeping score on self" (p. 14), and this theme is inherent in all of his work.

Drucker is perhaps best known for his philosophy on "management by objectives," which emphasizes the significance of planning, goals, and evaluating results against pre-established expectations. All of this clearly is management, but it is a crucial part of being an effective leader . . . namely, having a vision and evaluating, on a regular basis, the progress being made toward realizing the vision.

This book is easy to read and gives the reader a feeling that anyone can be whatever one wants to be. It also stresses the importance of making a difference in people's lives and not being remembered merely for writing a book or developing a theory. This book is good for helping individuals develop their leadership abilities.

Bennis, W. (1993). *An invented life: Reflections on leadership and change*. Reading, MA: Addison-Wesley.

This is a retrospective look by Bennis about his own life and work. He candidly explains leadership through his lens as a social scientist and business administrator, and offers thoughts on comparing leaders to managers: "I decided that the kind of university president I wanted to be was one who led, not managed. That's an important difference. Many an institution is well managed yet very poorly led. It excels in the ability to handle all daily routine inputs yet never asks whether the routine should be done in the first place" (p. 31). Bennis speaks of a democratic leadership style as what is most promoted in U.S. industry and defines it as including: "1) full and free communication, regardless of rank and power; 2) a reliance on consensus rather than on coercion or compromise to manage conflict; 3) the idea that influence is based on technical competence and knowledge rather than on the vagaries of personal whims or prerogatives of power; 4) an atmosphere that permits and even encourages emotional expression as well as task-oriented behavior; and 5) a basically human notion, one that accepts the inevitability of conflict between the organization and the individual but is willing to cope with and mediate this conflict on rational grounds." He ends with the importance of leaders of all organizations, small and large, to partner with others and collaborate in order to best set the stage for change.

Bennis, W. (2003). *On becoming a leader: Leadership classic—Updated and expanded,* (2nd Ed.). Reading, MA: Addison-Wesley.

Written by one of the foremost authorities on leadership, this book is a classic in the field. Beginning with the conviction that everyone can potentially be a leader, this book is a reflective exploration of the nature of this elusive phenomenon and the qualities and characteristics of those who serve as leaders. The author notes that after doing a Google search on "lack of leadership" he received more than 27,000 hits. He feels there are few leaders answering our nation's call for leaders, and he worries about the impact of this lack of leadership since "our quality of life depends on leaders" (p. 2). He gives many examples of where leadership is lacking in our world including American business and the Roman Catholic Church.

Although leadership can be provided by almost anyone, leaders are not ordinary people, according to Bennis. They work everywhere; they serve as guides; they take risks, and they fail. Leaders always learn from those failures; they engage in continuous learning and self-development, and they know themselves. Indeed, this author notes that leadership is a journey of personal development.

By using many examples—from Norman Lear to Gloria Steinem and from the executive director of the American Association of University Women to the chairman and CEO of Johnson & Johnson—Bennis helps the reader understand how leaders need to master the contexts in which they find themselves, create new contexts, use their instincts and intuition, and be innovators who help others move through chaos, among other things. These examples also are used to illustrate the differences between leadership and management.

Serious students of leadership will want this classic reference in their collection. It is insightful and offers many practical suggestions for developing as a leader. It is a welcome revision of his classic first edition.

Bennis, W., & Nanus, B. (1985). *Leaders. The strategies for taking charge.* New York: Harper & Row.

This is the seminal work in which the claim that "managers are people who do things right and leaders are people who do the right things" (p. 21) is first made. The authors speak to the dramatic changes taking place in our world and acknowledge the dire need for competent leadership and for "great flexibility and awareness on the part of leaders and followers alike" (p. 14).

Based on the results of a 2-year study of individuals who were thought to be leaders, Bennis and Nanus identified four major themes/areas of competency/"human handling skills" (p. 26) that emerged. Those strategies are as follows: attention through vision (i.e., creating a focus or having an agenda, particularly one that draws others in), meaning through communication (i.e., expressing ideas powerfully so that others understand and want to support them), trust through positioning (e.g., making one's position known, being reliable, and being "tirelessly persistent [with] relentless dedication," [p. 45]), and the deployment of self (i.e., having a positive self-regard, knowing one's strengths and weaknesses, and setting high goals). Each of these strategies is discussed thoroughly, and many ideas are offered as to how one can implement each.

The authors conclude by saying that we must "raise the search for new leadership to a national priority" (pp. 228–229). They urge the purposeful and continuous development of leaders because without effective leaders, the best our society can do is maintain the status quo; at worst, our society could disintegrate.

Bennis, W., Spreitzer, G., & Cummings, T. (2001). *The future of leadership: Today's top leadership thinkers speak to tomorrow's leaders.* San Francisco: Jossey-Bass.

This book is a collection of essays written in tribute to Warren Bennis for his distinguished life and career by present leaders (short bibliographies of whom are included in the book). It is divided into six parts: setting the stage for the future, organizations of the future, leaders of the future, how leaders stay on top of their game, insights from young leaders, and some thoughts on the leadership challenges of the next generation. Bennis also added to this book his thoughts on challenging issues that leaders must be able to understand and manage if they are to be successful in the future: how organizations collaborate, whether future leaders will be comparable to present leaders, whether employees will be calling all of the shots, how the inequalities of different people and organizations will affect leadership, demographics, what loyalty will exist between employees and organizations, what organizational change will ensue, personal and career balance, and where the new leaders will come from.

Bennis, W., & Thomas, W. (2002). *How eras, values, and defining moments shape leaders.* Boston: Harvard Business School Press.

This book is a compilation of ideas on leadership development and the generational differences between the Geeks (people under 30 years old) and the Geezers (people over 70 yrs old), which are basically most of the baby boomers and parents. The book focuses on the young and the old more so than on the people between 30 and 70 years of age. The leadership development model described in this book can help readers develop the four areas that these authors define as leadership: voice, integrity, adaptive capacity, and ability to engage others by creating a vision. A great emphasis is on what the authors call "crucible moments," which are life-changing experiences that people have throughout their lives and that call for leadership. This book is easy to read, worthwhile, and helpful to improve self-confidence and general self-concept regarding one's ability to achieve dreams and personal visions.

Bolman, L. G., & Deal, T. E. (2001). *Leading with soul: An uncommon journal of spirit (New & revised ed.).* San Francisco: Jossey-Bass.

Using the story of Steve, a dispirited leader in search of something more meaningful in his life than "the bottom line," these authors help the reader see and appreciate the spiritual dimensions of leadership and how work and spirit can and, in their opinion, need to be connected. They discuss the interrelationship of leaders and followers, the "gifts" of leadership (love, power, and significance), and the legacy of leadership. This book challenges the reader to look deep inside oneself and reflect on one's true self and values. Finally, the dialogue between the authors and an "interviewer" that concludes the book provides insights into why they examined the concept of the soul of leadership and how this work has affected individuals in various positions in diverse organizations.

Book, E. W. (2000). *Why the best man for the job is a woman.* New York: HarperBusiness.

This book reports on intensive studies the author conducted with 14 women who have exhibited leadership, primarily in the corporate world. Among the strengths that were common to all women were "a gravity-defying level of self-confidence . . . a preternatural sense of exactly what their [followers] want . . . [and a tendency to] foster a more collegial environment" (p. xiii). The author claims that "evidence is mounting that the style of leadership women offer is beneficial not only to employees but also to the bottom line, [perhaps because] women are better at communicating, empowering people and being positive" (p. xv).

The author provides extensive descriptions of the key characteristics of what she calls "new paradigm leadership": selling one's vision, reinventing the rules, having a laser focus to achieve, maximizing high touch in an era of high tech, turning challenge into opportunity, and having courage under fire. She contrasts these with features of the old paradigm—masculine, hierarchical, command-and-control oriented, opposed to change, focused on individual efforts, and limited to communication—and describes the advantages of new paradigm leadership.

In conclusion, Book offers a number of tips on becoming a new paradigm leader and encourages women to assume such roles with enthusiasm. As such, this book provides a thoughtful analysis of women's leadership styles and serves as a helpful guide to those wishing to integrate such styles into their own repertoire.

Burns, J.M. (1978). *Leadership.* New York: Harper Torchbooks.

This book is truly a classic! It was Burns who first acknowledged that "leadership is one of the most observed and least understood phenomenon on earth" (p. 2) and then proceeded to help us understand this complex concept.

He noted how little we knew at the time about leadership and how to develop it—despite the hundreds of definitions of the term!—and how little attention was given to the significance of followers and the "interwoven texture of leadership and followership" (pp. 4–5). He also analyzed the nature of power and the role of power in leadership, and explored the ways in which leaders help release the potentials of others.

In his attempt to clarify the meaning of leadership, Burns offers distinctions between *transactional* and *transformational* leadership, and introduces the notion of *moral* leadership. In recent years, many authors have "carried the banner" of transformation leadership, but Burns was the first to name it and describe it exquisitely.

As a result of Burns' seminal work on leadership, our understanding of this complicated concept has progressed enormously. This is a book that must be read as a foundation to subsequent works about leadership.

Burns, J. M. (2003). *Transforming leadership: A new pursuit of happiness*. New York: Atlantic Monthly Press.

In this book, Burns expands on his notion of transformational leadership. He asserts that "to transform something . . . is to cause a metamorphosis in form or structure, a change in the very condition or nature of a thing" (p. 24) . . . a change of breadth and depth.

The primary focus of this book is an examination of how a number of leaders in the past, including the American Founding Fathers, embraced and lived the three standards or norms that Burns claims constitute a good leader: virtue, ethics, and transforming values. He then conducts an extensive analysis of how these standards shaped the Declaration of Independence's emphasis on life, liberty, and the pursuit of happiness, with particular emphasis on the latter (hence, the book's subtitle).

While Burns offers many insightful comments about leaders, leadership, followers, empowerment, and other topics relevant to a study of leadership, they often are difficult to cull from the discussions of the pursuit of happiness. Leadership scholars will want to study this book carefully, but novices to leadership studies are likely to benefit more from other resources.

Chaleff, I. (1998). *The courageous follower: Standing up to and for our leaders*. San Francisco: Berrett-Koehler Publishers.

This book gets to the heart of what leadership truly is and how it grows from followership. The author describes followership in a very positive way and avoids the negative connotations often associated with being a follower.

Chaleff speaks to being an *effective* follower and how such individuals are critical to generating effective leaders. He offers many fundamental, common sense, helpful ideas that could be most useful to the person interested in empowering her/himself and others, creating a vision, making a change, and preparing for a leadership role.

The author makes a point of explaining the significance of being a follower, supporting the leader's vision, and participating actively in change processes. A major point made by Chaleff is that followers do not do things simply at the bidding of leaders, nor do they hide behind leaders. Instead, followers do things because they think those things are best for themselves and for the organization. Followers, according to Chaleff, are not weak or passive. They are dynamic and passionate about many issues.

This book is a "must read" for understanding the relationship between leaders and followers and for appreciating the significance of followers in making change and realizing visions.

Clampitt, P., & DeKoch, R. (2001). *Embracing uncertainty: The essence of leadership*. Armonk, NY: M. E. Sharpe.

The authors make the case that embracing uncertainty is more effective and rewarding than trying to eliminate it. They advocate that leaders recognize that they will never have all of the right answers and "not knowing" is quite legitimate. Leaders should never feel bad about not knowing but should attempt to foster this belief in their followers so increased creativity and increased morale is the outcome. *The Working Climate Survey* developed by these authors to measure one's tendency to embrace uncertainty provides fascinating insight to one's comfort with uncertainty and ambiguity. This tool is included in this book, along with directions for interpreting results, and it also is available online at *www.imetacomm.com/edu*, where one can get immediate feedback.

Cohen, W. (2004). *The art of the strategist: 10 essential principles for leading your company to victory*. New York: American Management Associates.

This book is a must-read for those wanting to learn new strategies of fulfilling a group's or individual's vision. It emphasizes the importance of being aware of environmental influences and recognizes that it sometimes is necessary to change strategy or components of strategy in order to fulfill goals. The fact that the success of a strategy depends on the "judgment and leadership qualities of the individual responsible for the undertaking" (p. vii) is the underlying premise.

Cohen offers 10 essential principles which are worth reading and pondering: commit fully to a definite objective; seize the initiative and keep it; economize to mass your resources; use strategic positioning; do the unexpected; keep thing simple; prepare multiple, simultaneous alternatives; take the indirect route to your objective; practice timing and sequencing; and exploit your success. The author then gives excellent realistic examples of both successful and unsuccessful strategizing and offers reasonable ideas of how to examine one's plan and make changes mid-stream so success is the outcome. Ideas for strategizing in an escalating crisis and in emergencies also are discussed.

Coleman, L., & Deal, T. (2001). *Leading with soul: An uncommon journey of spirit*. San Francisco: Jossey-Bass.

This book is definitely a must-read. It not only describes the search for soul and spirit, but it also shares the story of one man's search. In the capitalistic world we live in today, this book is a refreshing, wonderful experience. As the authors say, "we must reinforce the workplace with passion, zest, and spirit" (p. 6). They define soul as "personal and unique, grounded in depths of personal experience" (p. 9). Spirit is defined as "transcendent and all embracing; it is the universal source, the oneness of all things" (p.9). The authors explain how we need to relearn how to lead with soul, and they discuss how soul, spirit, and faith belong at the heart of leadership.

Coles, R. (2000). *Lives of moral leadership.* New York: Random House.

This book powerfully conveys the meaning of moral leadership using well-known and influential, as well as "ordinary," people as examples. The lives and work of individuals like Robert Kennedy, Gandhi, and Albert Jones, a Boston bus driver, are used to illustrate the bond that develops between true leaders and their followers, and how "moral energy" helps our society respond to crises and challenges. Coles asserts that "we need heroes, people who can inspire us, help shape us morally, spur us on to purposeful action" (p. xi), and he acknowledges that "from time to time we are called on to *be* those heroes, leaders for others, either in a small, day-to-day way, or on the world's larger stage" (p. xi). Reading this book helps one appreciate what moral leadership is and how it is achieved. As such, it is a most significant resource in today's environment.

Conger, J. (1992). *Learning to lead: The art of transforming managers into leaders.* San Francisco: Jossey-Bass.

Conger firmly believes that leadership can be "broken down" into specific behaviors, those behaviors can be taught, and they can be learned. In fact, this book is an account of the author's own experiences in learning to be a leader, specifically through his participation in the following innovative leadership development programs: Kouzes and Posner's Leadership Challenge, the Center for Creative Leadership's Leadership Development Program, the Experiential Pecos River Learning Center Program, and the Vision Quest Program.

The author explains the significance of leaders having a vision, being inspirational, demonstrating charisma, being empowered, and acting as a transformational change agent. He asserts that one can learn these skills.

Work experiences, taking advantage of opportunities that present themselves, educational advancement, mentors, and experiencing hardship, all are variables identified by Conger as fostering leadership. He explains the historical development of leadership training and points out the importance of having such programs focus on providing feedback to participants regarding their conceptual development, skill building, and personal growth.

Conger also explores some of the more "common" theories about leadership. He explains how situational leadership and the "task-versus-relationship" contingency model of the 1980s lack the strategic envisioning, inspirational speaking, and management of change that he feels is absolutely essential for an effective leader in today's environments. He believes that all aspiring leaders need to participate in the kind of personal growth programs that he discusses in this book.

Covey, S. (1991). *Principle-centered leadership*. New York: Summit Books.

This book is grounded in the idea that having principles to guide one's life, like a compass guides one's journey, makes for a more productive, fulfilling life. Covey presents his ideas regarding the principles of vision, leadership, and human relationships as the way to make decisions in one's personal, interpersonal, managerial, and organizational lives. He offers suggestions on how to cultivate eight characteristics that facilitate the making of what he calls a "principle-centered leader."

This excellent book on self-leadership can be used as a rich resource to assist others in their development as leaders, particularly "principle-centered" leaders. Covey's ideas center around the importance of a leader being a pathfinder—someone who can align an organization's or an individual's structure with an individual's behavior, **not** the organization's behavior—and a facilitator or empowerer of others. By pathfinder, Covey means being able to move an individual or group down a path or to realize a vision. The pathfinder is an individual who, by using leadership, moves individuals or organizations in new directions, an approach that is vastly different from making changes merely in response to revised organization policies and expectations.

Covey, S. (2006). *The 8th habit: From effectiveness to greatness*. New York: Running Book Press.

This book is an excellent sequel to *The 7 Habits of Highly Effective People*. The author has added the idea of "finding your voice and encouraging others to find theirs" as the 8th habit. He describes how all individuals can discover the voices that evolve from three gifts at birth: freedom to choose, natural laws, and the four intelligences (mental, physical, spiritual, and emotional). He gives multiple examples of how people can use these ideas to improve themselves and become more holistic people and leaders.

Covey discusses how leadership roles have changed and gives examples of how individuals can maximize their leadership skills with new roles. He also describes what he sees as new roles for leaders: modeling, path-finding, aligning, and empowering. He discusses the value of vision, discipline, passion, and conscience in leaders and gives many real-life examples for using the new roles of leadership. The book also offers advice on how a person can change from being a "want to" person to a "can do" person, and the section on Frequently Asked Questions about his ideas of leadership is helpful.

Denhardt, R., & Denhardt, J. (2006). *The dance of leadership: The art of leading in business, government, and society*. New York: M. E. Sharpe Inc.

This book emphasizes the need for each individual to lead, no matter what his/her role. The authors assert that each person should use his/her leadership ability to improve the work setting, home situation, or other circumstance. They offer a view of leadership that originates from the arts, noting that "artists see the world in a way quite different from others . . . they see the world in terms of an especially intense and textured interplay of space, time, and energy" (p. 6). Denhardt and Denhardt weave an interesting story about how one cannot really have a single operational definition of leadership, and they assert that "the only thing that really counts in leadership is that which you can't explain" (p.10).

This book is interesting and entertaining and challenges the reader to seriously think about the emotional aspects of leadership and the importance of the leader's audience (i.e., followers). The authors explore various concepts such as rhythms of human interaction, communication, spontaneity, and creativity; and they share their rendition of the difference between leadership and management. These authors make a strong argument that leadership originates from art, not science.

DePree, M. (1989). *Leadership is an art*. New York: Currency Doubleday.

This book is about "the art of leadership; liberating people to do what is required of them in the most effective and humane way possible" (p. 1). As an art, leadership is something one learns over time.

One of the most significant aspects of leadership, according to DePree, is a genuine concern for and about others. Leaders understand the diversity of the talents, gifts, and skills others possess and find ways to allow each individual to contribute to a cause or purpose in her/his own way.

The author asserts that leaders serve others—". . . they are stewards more than they are owners"—and they "should leave behind them assets and a legacy" (p. 13). They are responsible for identifying, developing, and nurturing future leaders, and they bind people together to accomplish great things. They provide and help to maintain the momentum of a group, and they keep the group focused on the values and visions that guide them.

This easy-to-read book includes many insightful points about leaders and leadership that stimulate one's thinking in new ways. The conceptualization of leadership as an art, but an art that can be learned, is a useful one for the would-be leader.

Dreher, D. (1996). *The Tao of personal leadership*. New York: HarperBusiness.

This book is a rich blend of the principle of centering and balancing one's life and the Taoist philosophy of engaging in compassion while remaining detached. It emphasizes the importance of realizing the power of living systems that generate energy all around us, and it reinforces the appreciation of all people potentially becoming leaders, regardless of their "station" in life.

Communication, team building, having an appetite for constant change, credibility, risk taking, and the ability to facilitate others in accomplishing goals/vision are necessary assets of a strong leader, according to Dreher. The author describes the Tao leader as being a pioneer, a pathfinder, a person who guides with intuition, someone who constantly faces the unknown with excitement, and someone who turns conflict into opportunities for stronger relationships, greater knowledge, and better solutions. The author has written an exhilarating account of how one can develop one's leadership capacity in exponential fashion.

Gardner, J. W. (1990). *On leadership*. New York: The Free Press.

John Gardner is one of the experts on the topic of leadership, and he reports, in this book, insights gained from a 5-year study of the phenomenon. He distinguishes leadership from management and expresses the great need we have for true leaders, individuals "who are exemplary, who inspire, who stand for something, [and] who help us set and achieve goals" (p. xi).

One of the most significant contributions Gardner makes through this book is helping the reader understand what he calls "the tasks of leadership." Included in those "tasks" are the following:

Envisioning Goals . . . pointing us in the right direction or asserting a vision

Affirming Values . . . reminding the group of the norms and expectations they share

Motivating . . . stimulating and encouraging others to act

Managing . . . planning, setting priorities, and making decisions

Achieving a Workable Unity . . . managing conflict and promoting unity within the group

Explaining . . . teaching followers and helping them understand why they are being asked to do certain things

Serving as a Symbol . . . acting in ways that convey the values of the group and its goals

Representing the Group . . . speaking on behalf of the group

Renewing . . . bringing members of the group to new levels

In fulfilling these tasks, leaders must work collaboratively with followers, whom Gardner refers to as constituents. He acknowledges that "followers often perform leader-like acts" (p. 23) and recognizes the significant role that followers play in accomplishing change and realizing a vision.

Finally, Gardner draws on the work of many researchers to identify several attributes of leaders, including the following: physical vitality and stamina (i.e., a high energy level), intelligence and judgment-in-action (i.e., ability to identify and solve problems, set priorities, etc.), willingness to accept responsibilities (i.e., exercise initiative, bear the burden of making a decision, and step forward when no one else will), task competence (i.e., knowing the task at hand and the system), understanding followers/constituents and their needs, skill in dealing with people, a need to achieve, the capacity to motivate others, and courage. He also discusses how leaders need to use power and how they need to be morally responsible.

Gladwell, M. (2005). *Blink: The power of thinking without thinking*. New York: Little, Brown.

Although this book is not about leadership *per se*, it nevertheless offers valuable insights for anyone who strives to fulfill the role of leader. It is a book about how we think without thinking and how this process can be very valuable or have disastrous consequences.

Gladwell notes that "our world requires that decisions be sourced and footnoted" (p. 52). He then challenges that approach and labels it a mistake, asserting that "if we are to learn to improve the quality of the decisions we make, we need to accept the mysterious nature of our snap judgments. We need to respect the fact that it is possible to know without knowing why we know" (p. 52).

While somewhat unorthodox, Gladwell's perspective is congruent with much of the leadership literature, which notes that leaders often rely on their intuition and do what they believe . . . in their hearts . . . is right. As such, the reader interested in developing her/himself as a leader could benefit from these ideas that help one see the world in a different way.

Goleman, D. (1998). *Working with emotional intelligence.* New York: Bantam Books.

This is an interesting book describing how emotions affect one's life even more than one's intelligence quotient. The author asks the question, "Have you known leaders who are smart and experienced, but failed because they could not form collaborative relationships?" Goleman says a leader must be a master of emotional intelligence, and leaders must build their relationships with commitment and empathy. He suggests that emotional intelligence influences one's success at home, work, and school, and it affects how people interact with others and work in teams. Goleman discusses how one can improve one's emotional intelligence and how it increases with age. Essentially this book explains how people can be more successful if they can deal with their own emotions, learn to work with other people's emotions, and respond appropriately to others.

A leader must be visionary and capable of getting people motivated to participate in new ideas, making change, and working in totally different ways than ever before. Goleman explains how having emotional intelligence will help leaders be successful in these and other areas.

Goleman, D., Boyatzis, R., & McKee, A. (2002). *Primal leadership.* Boston: Harvard Business School Press.

This book speaks to the concept of resonance, which is defined as "a reservoir of positivity that frees the best in people "(p. ix). The authors expand on this concept as they explain that at its root, the primal job of leadership is emotional. Being intelligent about emotions is extremely significant to leaders being successful, and the authors discuss how maximizing the power one derives from being emotionally intelligent improves performance. The relationship between neurotransmitters and mood is exciting to read, as it illustrates how leaders' moods affect their behavior and the behavior of those they lead.

Examples of how emotionally intelligent leaders are successful in guiding organizations during chaotic times are excellent and well worth reading. The leadership competencies of emotional intelligence—self-awareness, self-management, social awareness, and relationship management—are clearly explained, and the idea that "there are many leaders and not just one" (p. xiii) pervades the book.

Greene, R. (1998). *The 48 laws of power.* New York: Viking.

This author claims that "all of us hunger for power, and almost all of our actions are aimed at gaining it" (p. xix), and he asserts that "if the game of power is inescapable, better to be an artist than a denier or a bungler" (p. xix). Given these perspectives,

Greene then goes on to describe thoroughly 48 laws that, he claims, will help one attain and retain power. Among those laws are the following: conceal your intentions, learn to keep people dependent on you, keep others in suspended terror, play all the way to the end, and preach the need for change, but never reform too much at once.

It is obvious that these laws reflect a Machiavellian perspective on power, and the author fails to discuss more positive sources or uses of power. For those who find themselves in "cut-throat" environments where one must do anything to survive, these laws may be helpful. For those who aspire to providing leadership in the way it has been discussed in the *New Leadership Challenge: Creating the Future of Nursing* and proposed by most authorities on the subject, such actions will not empower followers, create a sense of unity, or renew leaders or followers. Perhaps reading this book serves as a good lesson in what *not* to do as a leader.

Grossman, S. (2006). *Mentoring in nursing: A dynamic and collaborative process.* New York: Springer.

This book is helpful for nurses who are interested in empowering others, be that in academic or healthcare settings. The author offers a new definition of mentoring in nursing that encompasses the multiple components of the mentoring process. Examples of various mentoring models are described, and perspectives of both mentors and mentees are shared.

Various tools to assist in developing mentoring are cited, along with precepting models and programs. The idea that young and old need to mentor each other in the nursing profession if the profession's covenant with the public is to be kept is reinforced.

Harvard Business Review on leadership. (1998). Cambridge, MA: Harvard Business School Press.

This collection of eight articles reflects some of the foremost thinkers in the area of leadership including Mintzberg, Kotter, and Zaleznik. Many of the articles are accompanied by an executive summary, and most are followed by a retrospective commentary by the author. Mintzberg, for example, even offers some self-study questions after his chapter.

Clearly, these writings are significant in that they raise key questions such as the following: Are managers and leaders different? What do leaders really do? How do chief executives really lead? Why is providing leadership difficult?

At the end of the text is a short paragraph describing all of the contributing authors and their accomplishments since their seminal pieces were originally published. This book is definitely "must reading" for those wishing to develop a comprehensive understanding of the complex phenomenon of leadership.

Hein, E. C. (Ed.). (1998). *Contemporary leadership behavior: Selected readings* (5th ed.). Philadelphia: Lippincott.

This book is a collection of articles that were originally published in a variety of journals. The articles are organized into categories that focus on the culture of nursing (e.g., caring and gender socialization), theories of leadership and attributes of leaders, leadership behaviors (e.g., assertiveness, advocacy, and mentoring), the organizational setting, and shaping nursing's future.

This is a good resource of varied articles and differing perspectives on topics relevant to leadership. Chapters can be read out of sequence, and no chapter depends on the preceding, thereby giving readers a great deal of flexibility in how to use the book.

NOTE: Previous editions of this book contain some of the same readings and some different ones. They also are helpful references. The publication dates of those editions are as follows: 1st, 1982; 2nd, 1986; 3rd, 1990; and 4th, 1994. E.C. Hein and M.J. Nicholson edited the first three editions.

Helgesen, S. (1990). *The female advantage: Women's ways of leadership.* New York: Doubleday Currency.

In this book, one of the few that deals specifically with women as leaders, Helgesen describes ways in which women lead differently than men. Based on a study of women leaders in the workplace, she found patterns of behaving and approaches to making decisions and setting priorities that were quite different from what had been reported in studies of male leaders.

Women in Helgesen's study were very concerned about being involved in the work of the organization, keeping relationships healthy and productive, making time for activities that were not directly related to their work (e.g., parenting responsibilities), and maintaining a "big picture" orientation. They also viewed their jobs as only one element of who they were, not as *the* factor that defined who they were, and they preferred to see themselves at the center of things, rather than at the top.

As a result of these values, perspectives and preferences, women tended to create operational structures that were more web-like rather than hierarchical. Such structures provide for more interaction among members of the group, allow for more participation of all players in goal setting and decision-making, and result in greater inclusion.

Helgesen views these differences in the ways women lead as great strengths, strengths that are having and will continue to have dramatic effects on the nature of our organizations. The book provides a provocative analysis of women leaders and the way they can use their different perspectives and values to change organizations.

Hesselbein, F., Goldsmith, M., & Somerville, I. (1999). *Leading beyond the walls.* San Francisco: Jossey-Bass.

This book, which is a collection of writings by leaders in the field of leadership, is a publication of the Drucker Foundation. It "explores what is needed to transcend the personal walls that inhibit effectiveness and the organizational, social, and political boundaries that inhibit reaching out, [and it calls upon leaders to] forge partnerships that are essential in the increasingly challenging period ahead" (p. xii). The authors acknowledge that each of us is surrounded by walls—walls of policy, procedures, assumptions, safety, familiarity, and security—but these walls that protect us also can "inhibit movement, limit understanding, restrict engagement, and diminish our relevance in the wider world" (p. 2). For these reasons, leaders are challenged to move beyond the walls that bind individuals, organizations, and institutions.

Among the strategies offered to help individuals lead beyond the walls are the following: be courageous, take risks, be passionate, trust in people, affirm our past but celebrate our present and future, "challenge the gospel" (p. 4), engage in long-term collaboration, create community, be aware of and be true to your core values, develop systems rooted in freedom of choice rather than in coercion and control, share information, and seek unity rather than competition. These and other themes are woven throughout this book and serve as guideposts for the would-be leader. As such, this book is a valuable resource for those wishing to fully understand this complex phenomenon.

Houser, B. P., & Player, K. N. (2007). *Pivotal moments in nursing: Leaders who changed the path of a profession, Volume II.* Indianapolis, IN: Sigma Theta Tau International.

This book spotlights 11 nurses who moved our discipline ahead in significant ways. Included among those studied are Mary Elizabeth Carnegie, Imogene King, Ruth Watson Lubic, and Margaret McClure. Each nurse was interviewed and her "history" analyzed, and from these analyses, the authors drew conclusions about leaders. Their work helps the reader appreciate how leaders meet and overcome barriers and challenges to the ideas they propose that are "out of the mainstream," how they use their high energy level and passion to keep moving forward, how they are willing to always "go the extra mile" for their colleagues and for the profession itself, and how they become politically astute to deal with influential people in their environments.

It is clear from the study of these nurse leaders that they viewed themselves as rebels and were comfortable with that role. In addition, each of the individuals spotlighted had a vision and was able to see a bigger picture than others were able to see. The book, therefore, helps define what leadership is and offers insights into how one develops as a leader.

NOTE: The first volume of this book was published in 2004. It followed a similar format but presented twelve different nurse leaders, including Joyce Clifford, Luther Christman, Vernice Ferguson, Rheba de Tornyay, and Claire Fagin, among others.

Jaworski, J. (1998). *Synchronicity: The inner path of leadership.* San Francisco: Berrett-Koehler.

This author calls on Jung's classic definition of synchronicity—"a meaningful coincidence of two or more events, where something other than the probability of chance is involved"—to discuss what he refers to as "the most subtle territory of leadership, creating the conditions for 'predictable miracles'" (p. ix). Thus begins this fascinating book that focuses on how leaders shape the future instead of simply responding to the present.

Jaworski notes that most contemporary institutions are leaderless and bemoans this state of affairs in light of his expressed belief that there is leadership potential in everyone. Using his own personal journey, he describes how "we can shape our future in ways that we rarely realize" (p. 9) and "participate in the unfolding process of the universe" (p. 44), not merely accept what comes our way. By facing and overcoming personal challenges (i.e., being afraid to step outside one's own narrow circle, being afraid to take the risk of stepping into the unknown, fearing that one cannot make a difference anyway), Jaworski responded to the "call to redefine what is possible, to see a vision of a new world and . . . undertake, step-by-step, what [was] necessary . . . to achieve that vision" (p. 58).

The personal journey described in this book helps the reader appreciate the risk-taking inherent in a leadership role, as well as the rewards of serving in such a role.

Joel Barker's leadershift: Five lessons for leaders in the 21st century. (1999). A Star Thrower film. Produced by AMI, St. Paul, MN.

This excellent video features Joel Barker, a futurist, who discusses how leaders build bridges between today and tomorrow and who asserts that the most important role of a leader is to find, recognize, and secure the future. Barker notes that the foundations to "building bridges" include trust, communication, and confidence, all of which are qualities of leaders as described by other experts. Armed with these qualities, leaders can and must exist at all levels and in all endeavors. In other words, leadership is no longer about privilege . . . instead, it is about responsibility.

Through a dynamic video that captures the attention of the viewer, Barker talks about the need for new paradigms, since they are the things that drive fundamental change in our organizations and society. He offers the following five "lessons" for the 21st century, all of which are wise words of counsel for anyone assuming a leadership role in the coming years: focus the majority of your efforts on the future, understand the nature of fundamental change, appreciate complex systems and how they work, examine your leadership style to see how it affects productivity, and create shared vision to build bridges to the future.

This video (accompanied by a PowerPoint presentation on a CD-ROM, a participant workbook, and a facilitator's guide) is an excellent resource in helping one understand the need for dramatic change in our ways of thinking and behaving if we are to make needed change and provide much-needed leadership.

Kelley, R. E. (1992). *The power of followership: How to create leaders people want to follow and followers who lead themselves.* New York: Doubleday Currency.

Robert Kelley presents one of the best discussions of followership that is available in the literature. His goal in writing this book was to "shift the spotlight toward follower-ship as *the* important phenomenon to study if we are to understand why organizations succeed or fail" (p. 5), and he achieves that goal extremely well.

This author talks about the increasing emphasis on teams and collaboration and the kind of power that followers can and do have in groups and organizations. He notes that "followers determine not only if someone will be accepted as a leader but also if that leader will be effective" (p. 13), and he asserts that effective followers are critical for success.

The term "effective follower" is not used lightly in this book. Indeed, Kelley describes five different followership styles: passive, conformist, pragmatist, alienated, and exemplary/effective. He offers ways to help the reader identify her/his followership style, argues for the importance of developing one's followership skills, and offers very convincing arguments why we should become followers.

This book, therefore, is unique in its attention to a critical, but frequently ignored role in the leadership process. It is one that must be read to gain a better appreciation of the concept of followership.

Koestenbaum, P. (2002). *Leadership: The inner side of greatness* (2nd ed.). San Francisco: Jossey-Bass.

This book is a philosophical analysis of individuals and what it takes for successful leaders to achieve specific goals. It is not a synthesis of stories about people who have been successful but rather a compilation of how to create environments and societies that will facilitate the achievement of goals. Koestenbaum describes his Leadership Diamond Model, which revolves around the concepts of time, democracy, motivation, teamwork, and salesmanship.

This is a good book to read if one wishes to analyze one's leadership ability and/or develop one's leadership skills. There are some excellent cases, such as the Enron scandal, that examine marketing morale and history, and the exercises and checklists to assist the reader in leadership development are helpful.

Kouzes, J. M. & Posner, B. Z. (1993). *Credibility: How leaders gain and lose it . . . Why people demand it.* San Francisco: Jossey-Bass.

The purpose of this book is to explore, in depth, the quality that makes for a leader con-stituents (i.e., followers) would want to follow: credibility. Based on extensive research, the authors conclude that people have very high expectations of their leaders, wanting them to "hold to an ethic of service, [be] genuinely respectful of the intelligence and contributions of their constituents, [and] put principles ahead of politics and other people before self-interests" (p. xvii).

Kouzes and Posner view leadership as a relationship and a service, with credibility clearly at its foundation. This book examines leadership as a relationship, talks about the benefits of credibility, and discusses the behaviors that convey and establish credibility. Among those behaviors are the following: knowing yourself and your values, appreciat-ing the strengths and talents of followers, reinforcing shared values, developing others to reach their fullest potential, making meaning out of the work or tasks to be done, and sustaining hope in the followers. How leaders develop/gain and can lose credibility also are discussed.

This analysis stimulates the reader to thoughtfully reflect on her/his own actions and how they establish or undermine credibility. Although other writers imply the significance of credibility in the leader/follower relationship, Kouzes and Posner make a most valuable contribution to our understanding of how leaders can be most effective by their careful study of the concept. Any discussion of leadership would be incomplete without a discussion of credibility; this book, therefore, is an excellent resource for enhancing such understanding.

Kouzes, J., & Posner, B. (1999). *Encouraging the heart: A leader's guide to rewarding and recognizing others.* San Francisco: Jossey-Bass.

The main theme in this book is that people who are recognized for their good work and encouraged are more likely to achieve higher levels of success. The authors recommend how leaders can "support the basic human need to be appreciated for what we do and who we are" (p. xii). They explain "encouraging the heart" with four ideas: leaders must follow general principles that reward people for work well done; leaders will not be perceived as being "soft" for encouraging the heart; leaders have multiple methods they use to encourage the heart; and all leaders must be aware of the soul and spirit involved in any organization. This is a good book for all to read, especially when the organizations in which we function appear to be losing their edge and failing to be responsive to all those involved in the work of the organization. This book gives the reader ideas on how to "keep hope alive" (p. xix).

Kouzes, J., & Posner, B. (1995). *The leadership challenge: How to keep getting extraordinary things done in organizations* (2nd ed.). San Francisco: Jossey-Bass.

This second edition of an excellent book reflects the authors' observations of what leaders do to encourage extraordinary accomplishments when they are leading, not managing. Their classic "five sets of behavioral practices" and "ten behavioral commitments" are described fully, and the importance of leaders having perseverance, having direction, empowering others, being role models, and recognizing others' contributions are all discussed thoroughly.

The book points out that leadership is a skill that can be developed by coaching and through experiential learning. The necessity of purposefully developing one's leadership is advanced, as is the notion that leadership is more important today than ever before if we are to achieve success in the future. The authors remind us that leadership is everyone's business and, therefore, everyone should accept the leadership "challenge" on a daily basis.

Kritek, P. (1994). *Negotiating at an uneven table: A practical approach to working with difference and diversity.* San Francisco: Jossey-Bass.

This book relates important lessons to people who want to be involved in decisions being made in an organization. It gives sound advice as well as good examples of how to negotiate conflicts, especially when the players are not "equal," and hints to assist the reader in being able to recognize when there is an uneven table are discussed. Conflict resolution or management is the theme of this book and the author applies it to nursing situations. The author addresses the inequalities and diversity with her "ten ways of being," which are helpful in opening one's mind to creative ways of managing conflict.

Leadership in Nursing. (1994). *Holistic Nursing Practice, 9*(1), entire issue.

This journal issue offers a thoughtful collection of articles about the nature of leadership, particularly as it relates to nursing. It is a useful resource since each article can be read independently of the others. The articles focus on many significant areas, all of which facilitate an understanding of the complex nature of leadership. Included among those areas are the following: the nature of leadership and ways to conceptualize it that make sense for 21st century practice; the holistic nature of leadership; transformational leadership, particularly as it relates to women leaders; the significance of followers; ethical aspects of leadership; the preparation of leaders; an exploration of the leadership that is needed to shape a preferred future for nursing; and an analysis of ten years of nursing leadership research.

All the articles in this issue are intended to "provide new insights and to explore important issues related to leadership" (p. vi). They accomplish that goal in a stimulating way that has relevance for our profession.

Lowney, C. (2003). *Heroic leadership: Best practices from a 450-year-old company that changed the world.* Chicago: Loyola Press.

This book was written by an individual who lived for 7 years as a Jesuit seminarian then moved into the corporate world, namely JP Morgan. This book uses what the author learned about the Jesuits (the 450-year-old company referred to in the book's subtitle) as a model for understanding leadership. It is exceptionally well written and presents many insightful ideas that focus on true leadership.

From his experience at JP Morgan, the author concluded that "It was clear that only a handful of banks would emerge as winners in our changing, consolidating industry. And the winners likely would be those whose employees could take risks and innovate, who could work smoothly on teams and motivate colleagues, and who could not only cope with change but also spur change. In short, *leadership* would separate winners from losers." (p. 3)

Throughout this fascinating, informative, and historically grounded book, the author highlights numerous examples of true leadership and illustrates the concepts most effectively. This book is highly recommended for those who wish to learn about leadership from a nontraditional source, as well as for those who wish to learn more about "those radical Jesuits."

Malloch, K., & Porter-O'Grady, T. (2005). *Quantum leadership: Applications for the new world of work.* Sudbury, MA: Jones and Bartlett Publishers.

This book describes how leadership can be understood using quantum mechanics. Ideas that leaders can use to develop themselves and their followers are explained using various technological innovations while integrating the personal touch. The purpose of the book is to depict how leaders can be courageous and assist others by coaching for achievement, eliminating toxic behaviors, and having a future-perspective. A great emphasis of the authors is to delineate the significance of organizations having quantum-age characteristics such as being multilateral, multidirectional, relational, interacting, intersecting, and integrating. The book focuses on the "fully engaged leader" who is defined as someone with competence and intelligence, someone who is engaged in her/his work and other aspects of life, and someone who is conscious of his/her own and others' feelings. The case studies and scenarios offered in this book relate specifically to healthcare and are particularly helpful to the nurse or nursing student reader.

Marshall, S. P. (2006). *The power to transform: Leadership that brings learning and schooling to life.* San Francisco: Jossey-Bass.

This book focuses on the need for change in education and the kind of leadership that is needed to create a "new landscape for deep and integral learning" (pp. xi–xii). Such leadership is critical, Marshall notes, because "how we engage the minds of our children in learning profoundly shapes the patterns of their thinking and their thinking shapes the world" (p. xvii). Thus, one could conclude that the development of future leaders who think broadly and in innovative ways and who can help society create preferred futures is at stake if our education systems do not change.

This is an incredibly powerful book that should be read by all those involved in the educational process. It challenges long-held assumptions, presents challenges that must be taken up by leaders, and provides insight about the kind of leaders needed to transform education.

McCall, M. W. (1998). *High flyers: Developing the next generation of leaders.* Boston: Harvard Business School Press.

The major emphasis in this book is on corporate executives who have a "bent" toward management more so than leadership. Despite this emphasis, however, McCall presents many interesting ideas about leaders and what needs to be done to prepare individuals to be effective in those roles.

The author asserts that "organizations not only overlook people with the potential to develop but also frequently and unintentionally derail the talented people they have identified as high flyers by rewarding them for their flaws, teaching them to behave in ineffective ways, reinforcing narrow perspectives and skills, and inflating their egos" (p. xi). He notes that we often keep people from developing their full potential as leaders and, as a result, neither they nor their organizations progress as much as they otherwise could.

McCall firmly believes that leadership can be learned and points out that "the development of leaders is itself a leadership responsibility" (p. xii). Learning leadership, he says, is a "lifelong journey, with its lessons taught by the journey itself" (p. 17). He challenges each of us—as aspiring leaders who must take responsibility for our own growth, and as practicing leaders who must take responsibility for the leadership development of others—to attend to the conscious development of ourselves and others as leaders.

McFarland, L., Senn, L., & Childress, J. (1994). *21st century leadership: Dialogues with 100 top leaders*. New York: The Leadership Press.

This book is the result of collaboration among members of two associations—Leadership into the Next Century and the Senn-Delaney Leadership Consulting Group—that set out to identify the foremost thinking about leadership for the 21st century. The authors interviewed 100 of the most prominent leaders of the world (individuals from business, government, education, and other key sectors of society) and asked them for recommendations and ideas about how individuals and organizations could make their visions become realities in the new millennium.

The authors offer numerous ideas on how to be a successful risk taker, how to welcome change, why it is important to be flexible and adaptable, and how to create a vision that is achievable. They also speak to the importance of being globally aware, involved in networking, and connected to information of every conceivable type.

After reading this book one comes away realizing that it is impossible to strategically plan every step of one's professional or personal life. What is important and possible, however, is to become part of the dynamic change by partnering with others and continuously reaching for new growth.

Meyerson, D. E. (2001). *Tempered radicals: How people use difference to inspire change at work*. Boston: Harvard Business School Press.

"'Tempered radicals' are people who want to succeed in their organizations yet want to live by their values or identities, even if they are somehow at odds with the dominant culture of their organizations. Tempered radicals want to fit in *and* they want to retain what makes them different. They want to rock the boat, and they want to stay in it" (p. xi). So begins this fascinating book about those who walk the fine line between (a) resisting the majority culture and becoming an outcast for not being part of the team, and (b) wanting to fit in but not wanting to "sell out" on their values and principles.

Meyerson conducted interviews with more than 250 individuals in several different organizations, people who were seen as change agents. These individuals continued to operate in environments where their values were sometimes in conflict with those of the organization while they effected slow, incremental change in their organizations to achieve a closer alignment between personal and organizational values.

The author asserts that tempered radicals' acts "represent a crucial form of leadership, what [she] call[s] 'everyday leadership'" (p. xix). She describes why people act as tempered radicals, the many ways people may be different from their colleagues or co-workers, and how quiet resistance can lead to significant change. These discussions are most helpful to those who would aspire to be leaders in their organizations because they help one realize that change can come from within and that organizations can be altered to align with the values of the individuals who comprise them.

Nanus, B. (1992). *Visionary leadership: Creating a compelling sense of direction for your organization.* San Francisco: Jossey-Bass.

This is an excellent book about the concept of vision and its importance in the leadership process. Nanus asserts that vision is the key to leadership and without it, an individual cannot be considered a leader, nor can significant progress be made in our organizations, professions, or societies.

A leader, Nanus explains, must be attuned to the external environment (perhaps more so than the internal one) and be focused on the future, not merely on the present. This kind of direction-setting is what vision is all about, and it is what "attracts commitment and energizes people" (p. 16). Vision also serves to create meaning in the lives of the followers and establish a standard of excellence.

In addition to discussing what vision is, Nanus also helps the reader understand what vision is not. It is not, he says, prophesy, a mission, factual, true or false, static, or a constraint on actions. Instead, it is a view of the future that arises from one's values, passions, dreams, hopes, and desire to create a better world (or piece of the world).

Nanus offers many realistic and helpful strategies for how leaders can develop a compelling vision for the future of their organizations or groups. He also helps the reader think about ways to implement the vision.

Pandya, M., & Shell, R. (2005). *Lasting leadership: What you can learn from the top 25 business people of our times.* Philadelphia: Wharton School Publishing.

The Nightly Business Report (NBR), the most watched daily business program on television in the United States, collaborated with these authors to identify the most influential business leaders in the last 25 years. Some of the leaders include Mary Kay, John Bogle, Warren Buffett, Peter Drucker, Steven Jobs, Sam Walton, and Oprah Winfrey.

This book is a compilation of each of these leaders' business ventures, their leadership skills and styles, and the results or impact of their efforts. Reading how various leaders reacted, planned proactively, and learned from their success and mistakes is inspiring, and the attributes they identified as portraying lasting leadership are most helpful. Those attributes are as follows: "building a strong corporate culture, truth telling, finding and catering to under-served markets, 'seeing the invisible' (i.e., spotting potential winners or faint trends before their rivals or customers do), using price to build competitive advantage, managing and building their organization's brand (which, in some cases, may be their own name), being fast learners, and managing risk" (p. xx).

The authors noted that no one leader possessed all of these attributes, but each of the 25 leaders studied had more than one of these characteristics. This is a good book to learn how to develop and use one's talents at leading.

Porter-O'Grady, T., & Malloch, K. (2007). *Quantum leadership: A resource for health care innovation* (2nd ed.). Sudbury, MA: Jones and Bartlett Publishers.

The second edition of this book is directed toward individuals wanting to develop their own leadership skills and that of others, particularly leaders in healthcare who wish to maximize the leadership abilities of others in this era of transformation. The authors present their idea of how quantum mechanics is applied to human dynamic behavior and give useful examples of how important this idea is to successful organizations. There also are descriptions of how complexity theory, emotional competence, and transformational theories affect healthcare organizations. Examples of how to deal with "toxic" people in organizations are helpful, as are the ideas presented about how to apply successful conflict management strategies.

Robinson-Walker, C. (1999). *Women and leadership in health care: The journey to authenticity and power.* San Francisco: Jossey-Bass.

This book reports on intensive dialogue with nearly 100 women and men responsible for managing a significant portion of America's health care. It is clear that "women are simply not present in the numbers we would expect, nor do they ascend at the rate we would expect to the most senior leadership roles in health care" (p. ix). Given this reality, the author—who co-created the national Center for Nursing Leadership in the late 1990s— examines the significance of gender in the 21st century; stumbling blocks faced by women in reaching "the top"; and relationships among gender, values, and leadership.

The author asserts that the characteristics most commonly exhibited by women, particularly women interviewed for this book, are precisely the qualities needed by those providing leadership in health care: an ability to tolerate ambiguity, a collaborative style, dispersed power, consensus building, integrity, "doing the right thing—even when the price is high" (p. 185), and others. She then offers a number of "antidotes" to help women be more effective leaders: defusing gender's role in conflict, negotiations and power; using communication as a bridge; renewing our careers; nurturing ourselves; and mentoring others.

While this book acknowledges the difficulties women often have with taking on the leader role, it also is positive and offers specific strategies to overcome those difficulties. As such, it is an excellent resource on gender issues related to leadership.

Rosenbach, W. E., & Taylor, R. L. (Eds.). (2001). *Contemporary issues in leadership* (6th ed.). Boulder, CO: Westview Press.

This book (and all previous editions) is one of the best collections of readings about leadership. None of the articles—many of which have been published originally elsewhere, and several of which are classics in the field—has focused specifically on nursing (to date), but each of them offers many rich ideas that could easily be applied to a nursing context. The new edition offers readings divided into five sections: the human heart of leadership, leadership legacies, the follower factor, learning to lead, and leadership as a paradox. The book, therefore, continues to be a most valuable one for students and teachers of nursing.

This book draws on experts in various areas and includes original articles as well as ones previously published in the *Harvard Business Review, Leader to Leader, World Futures,* the *Wall Street Journal,* and *Compass: A Journal of Leadership.* It is, therefore, exciting and inclusive of diverse perspectives. Although several of the articles are from management journals, they clearly are focused on leadership, and this is one of the things that makes this collection of reading so valuable—it does not confuse management and leadership.

NOTE: All previous editions of this book also are quite valuable and include collections of different readings. The 1st edition was published in 1984, the 2nd in 1989, the 3rd in 1993, the 4th in 1998, and the 5th in 2001.

Schiff, K. G. (2005). *Lighting the way: Nine women who changed modern America.* New York: Hyperion.

Written by the daughter of former Vice President Al Gore, this book chronicles how nine extraordinary women worked behind the scenes and against the odds in the major political movements of the last century. It tells powerful stories of women who influenced women's suffrage, the decision to enter World War II, the struggle for civil rights, environmental health, the AIDS crisis, and other significant issues of the last 100 years.

In telling these stories, Schiff points out that women have always been consequential, if often unrecognized, political leaders and have been responsible for many of the most creative ideas that helped shape history. This book is uplifting and powerful, and is an excellent resource for the study of women as leaders.

Senge, P. (2006). *The fifth discipline: The art and practice of the learning organization* (2nd ed.). New York: Currency Doubleday.

This new edition of Senge's seminal work, *The Fifth Discipline,* describes how many of his ideas regarding leadership and management have been operationalized in organizations since the original 1990 publication. He shares the outcomes of his interviews with people from companies such as Intel, Ford, BP and HP, as well as organizations such as The World Bank, Roca, and Oxfam. Some new and particularly interesting chapters in this edition are *"Impetus,"* which describes how to build learning-oriented cultures instead of staying in one's comfort zone, *"Leaders' New Work,"* and *"Frontiers for the Future."*

Through this book, Senge teaches the reader how to see things differently (e.g., seeing the forest and the trees), how to deal with the constant struggle of being tugged by personal **and** work issues, and how to maximize one's creativity. This is perhaps a more management-focused book, but since being a good manager serves to strengthen one's leadership ability, it is a valuable resource.

Sinetar, M. (1998). *The mentor's spirit: Life lessons on leadership and the art of encouragement.* New York: St. Martin's Press.

This book is another excellent publication by the best-selling author of the following books: *Do What You Love . . . The Money Will Follow* and *To Build the Life You Want, Create the Work You Love: The Spiritual Dimension of Entrepreneuring.* It discusses the art of encouragement, which is the word Sinetar uses to mean mentoring. She describes 12 lessons of mentoring, explains how one can be mentored and how one can mentor others, and offers realistic strategies and easy-to-follow plans for both mentors and mentees.

This must-read book is easy to read, and it encourages the reader to want to be involved in a mentor-mentee relationship. Sinetar's main point, which constantly echoes throughout the book, is that no matter what one might think, a single person is not the center of the world . . . it really is much more worthwhile to reach out to, network with, encourage, and mentor others.

Soder, R. (2001). *The language of leadership.* San Francisco: Jossey-Bass.

The author suggests that management is a larger, more encompassing concept than leadership; however, he goes on to say that "This book deals with elements of leadership as applied to those in elected and other public offices . . . and those in the private sector" (p. xv), meaning, largely, that the focus is on individuals in management positions.

The author asserts that persuasion is "a critical aspect of leadership" (p. 3) and focuses most of the book on an analysis of the concept of persuasion and how leaders can use it to get others to do what they want. In addition, the author makes leadership seem like little more than political maneuvering (p. 28), almost as if one needs to be quite Machiavellian (e.g., use devious means to get information) in order to be successful as a leader. These perspectives are contradictory to most other literature on leadership.

In addition, the author seems to want to "impress" the reader with his knowledge of a wide range of literature by inserting quotes and "snippets" from various philosophers, historical figures, etc. A few such quotes and examples are helpful to illustrate a point, but after a while, it seemed that the author was inserting such items simply to impress the reader. Instead of accomplishing this goal, however, this style may obfuscate the real point of the book.

Spears, L. (Ed.). (1998). *The power of servant leadership: Essays by Robert Greenleaf.* San Francisco: Berrett-Koehler Publishers.

This book captures the vision and writings of the late Robert K. Greenleaf, who was the first to use the term "servant-leadership." According to Greenleaf, "servant-leadership" is a way of leading that puts serving others (e.g., customers, patients, employees) first. This collection includes the following eight essays written by Greenleaf throughout his career: *Servant-Leadership: Retrospect and Prospect, Education and Maturity, The Leadership Crisis, Have You a Dream Deferred?, The Servant as Religious Leader, Seminary as Servant, My Debt to E. B. White,* and *Old Age: The Ultimate Test of Spirit.*

All of the essays in this collection reflect Greenleaf's ideas about spirit, commitment to vision, and wholeness. Given this focus, this is a most reflective book that leaves the reader with a feeling of "wanting to do things right."

Spears. L. C. (Ed.). 1995. *Reflections on leadership: How Robert K. Greenleaf's theory of servant-leadership influenced today's top management thinkers.* New York: John Wiley & Sons.

This collection of 27 essays—written by some of the leading thinkers and practitioners of servant-leadership—brings together into one volume some of the most significant ideas about the concept and the growing influence of Robert K. Greenleaf's legacy. It begins with several chapters by Greenleaf himself, describing the evolution of his thinking and the development of his "theory."

This book is an excellent source of information about servant-leadership and how a variety of people have interpreted and lived the concept. It is inspiring and uplifting, and helps one think about leadership in a different way.

Staub, R. E. (1996). *The heart of leadership.* Provo, UT: Executive Excellence Publishing.

This comprehensive book provides step-by-step advice on how to develop effective leadership skills, as well as skills for becoming a productive follower. The author advocates the following practices of leadership: provide guidance through shared vision, focus on purpose, create followership, set standards while eliciting goals, read and understand others, provide resources, liberate motivation, support others, provide feedback, practice principled flexibility, solicit personal feedback, and cultivate the heart of courage.

Staub is a strong believer in everyone working together to lead an organization or group, not just one or two leaders "at the top." Reading this book reaffirms the notion, expressed by so many other experts on leadership, that true leadership is possible for everyone who can master her/his attitudes, express her/his ideas, and act on her/his dream(s).

Vance, C. (1979). Women leaders: Modern day heroines or social deviants? *Image,* *11*(2), 37-41.

Although nearly 30 years old, this article is worth reading. It talks about how women who provide leadership often are seen as social deviants . . . individuals who fail to follow the norms of society, who fail to "stay in their place," and who seem to want to take on male roles. Such ideas can still be found in our organizations today, thereby making the notion of "deviant" still relevant.

Vance's discussion of how risk taking and genuine leadership can be seen negatively alerts the reader to the need for personal strength, clarity of vision, and commitment in those who will be leaders. While some may see leaders as heroines, others see them as power hungry people who want to control others and create their own world. Thus, the would-be leader must be prepared to take on the challenge, find ways to develop collaborative relationships with followers, and persevere in pursuing one's vision and turning it into reality.

Vance, C., & Olson, R.K. (1998). *The mentor connection in nursing.* New York: Springer.

This book is not presented as a "leadership" book, but the nature of its focus— mentoring—makes it quite relevant in any study of leadership and followership. In addition, the book is one strategy used by these authors to realize their own vision of nurses mentoring each other. Its roots were in the 1977 and 1984 doctoral dissertations of the two authors, and it crystallized over more than a decade of collaboration between the two.

Mentoring, these authors say, is a unique type of developmental relationship. It involves colleagues helping each other grow and learn. It empowers each person in the relationship. It is a means to "strengthen the profession by ensuring an adequate supply of competent practitioners and leaders" (p. 3). As such, mentoring must become a natural part of the practice of all nurses.

Through the use of personal "stories," many of nursing's accomplished leaders help the reader understand the nature of mentoring, the value of such relationships, and the relevance of mentoring to nursing. A variety of contributing authors talk about negotiating the mentor relationship, peer mentoring, the privilege and responsibility of mentoring, mentoring in the practice and the academic setting, and global and cross-cultural mentoring. Many of these discussions incorporate personal experiences and are, therefore, particularly moving, meaningful, and memorable.

This is an excellent resource for understanding the phenomenon of mentoring. It also is a valuable collection of personal stories that present a positive view of our profession and that serve as "anchors" for neophytes who are looking for or hoping for a mentoring relationship. It is, in essence, an informative and an inspiring book.

Ward, M. (2001). *Beyond chaos: The underlying theory behind life, the universe, and everything.* New York: Thomas Dunce Books.

This book is an interesting discussion about the phenomenon of universality, or how physics explains "how inert lumps of matter conspire and self-organize to produce life" (p. ix). The book title is a bit lofty perhaps since, of course, one book cannot answer the underlying theory behind life, the universe, and everything! It does, however, present an excellent discussion of how patterns emerge in various systems, it is helpful in understanding chaos theory, and it is applicable to how organizations and individuals lead their organizations or professions through tumultuous times.

Wheatley, M. (2006). *Leadership and the new science: Discovering order in a chaotic world* (3rd ed.). San Francisco: Berrett-Koehler Publishers.

This third edition of Wheatley's seminal work on the New Science reinforces ideas presented initially in 1992 and offers many new ideas to challenge our thinking. Contrary to the scientific or Newtonian model of step-by-step planning, the New Science emphasizes the importance of exploring and accepting things the way they occur, as viewed from the perspectives of quantum physics, chaos theory, and biology.

Wheatley speaks to how leaders and those responsible for running organizations can benefit from application of the New Science. She asserts that by moving toward holism and appreciating the intricate relationships that exist between and among all things, one can develop and effectively use methods to change how people act, how they work, and how they view life. As a result of this interconnectedness between every single thing in the world [actually everything *plus* the world, according to Wheatley], every moment of one's day is dynamic and unpredictable. She emphasizes the importance of relationships, even at the subatomic level. Also, the idea that change and chaos are the most significant way to transform positively is integrated throughout the book. This edition offers examples of how self-organizing networks can flourish in our new world, and it presents information on how best to respond to disasters and stop terrorism. The author concludes that the fundamental work of this time centers around all of us discovering new ways of working and being together.

Wheatley explains how order and chaos can be seen as identical images and how these two seemingly opposite forces actually drive each other. Using natural phenomena (such as the evolution of the Grand Canyon, a babbling brook, and stormy weather), Wheatley creates complexity from simplicity and excites the reader with ideas of how the future will evolve from the whole, rather than from the parts. This is a "must-read" book for anyone interested in learning more about chaos theory and the New Science.

Wheatley suggests people organize their own "Leadership & the New Science" discussion groups by going to *www.bkconnection.com* or joining the listserv group.

Wheatley, M., & Kellner-Rogers, M. (1996). *A simpler way*. San Francisco: Berrett-Koehler.

This book offers a way of thinking about life in a dynamic and totally different way, and it is critical reading for those who wish to better understanding the New Science of Leadership. The authors share a magnificent collection of photographs of life, poems that convey the importance of being oneself, and narratives about simpler ways of viewing what the majority of people define as a stress-filled, non-enjoyable life.

This is a remarkable book about how to view life within the vastness of the universe. The authors speak to how life "self-organizes" without our planning every minute of every day, and how this organization creates our identities. The advantages of seeing the world self-organize without human manipulation is challenged, and ways to foster more creativity, freedom, and "real" meaning in life are generated. In addition, the notions of play, organization, self, emergence, and coherence are explored.

Yudkowsky, M. (2005). *The pebble and the avalanche: How taking things apart creates revolutions*. San Francisco: Berrett-Kohler.

The basic premise in this book is that revolutions—in how we think, how we do business, how we use technology, and so on—can be relatively easy to create by taking things apart, a process the author calls *disaggregation*. Disaggregation and innovation, the author asserts, have positive results such as heightened creativity in organizations, healthy competition, cost reduction, greater simplicity and synergy, all of which "sweep aside old infrastructures" (p. 22).

The notions of taking things apart and questioning basic premises or assumptions are valuable ways to stimulate change, and they can be helpful to leaders. In addition, the idea that a small change can trigger a huge avalanche of change has merit to the leader who attempts to influence complex, tradition-laden systems. This book, however, suggests that revolutionary change is relatively easy to achieve, which is a conclusion that must be questioned.

Zaleznik, A. (1977). Managers and leaders: Are they different? *Harvard Business Review, 55*(3), 67–78.

This article is must reading. It is one of the earliest works in which leadership is clearly distinguished from management and, as such, it is a classic in the field.

Zaleznik talks about the differences between managers and leaders in terms of how they relate to other people, to the organization, and to goals. He explores the different conceptions of work, different perspectives on solitary activity, and different views about conflict and status quo held by leaders and managers. For purposes of illustration, the author talks abut leaders and managers in the extreme, but he does acknowledge that managers can also be leaders and leaders also can be managers.

This article is clearly written and is extremely helpful in clarifying the distinctions between these two related phenomena. It is an essential reading in one's quest to understand leadership.

Index

Note: Page numbers followed by f refer to figures (illustrations); page numbers followed by t refer to tables.

Academic aids, to leadership, 158–162
to nursing, 146, 148
Academic excellence, 187
Accreditation bodies, in nursing, recommendations of, 148
Action-related differences, between leadership and management, 6t
Active/passive parameters, of followership, 42f
Activity-related differences, between leadership and management, 6t
Adversities, vs. possibilities, 118
Affirmation, of values, 4, 48
Aging population, healthcare needs of, 143
Alienated followers, 41
Allen, Paul, 78
Alpha leadership, 102
American Academy of Nursing, 161
American Nurses Foundation, 161
Androgynous leadership, 106, 107t. See also Gender perspectives, in leadership.
Antioch University, 158
Apprenticeship, 50. See also Followership.

Assessment tool(s), for creativity, 90, 94–96
for followership, 56–57
for leadership, 16–20
for leadership development, 166t
for readiness to change, 126, 131f–133f
Attention, personal, 12
Authenticity, 62
Authority, position of, 3, 7, 188
Avoidance, of conflict, 129

Bagley, D., 92
Balanced Budget Act (1997), 147
Beta leadership, 102
Biosphere, 118
Brain functions, left-sided, 87
right-sided, 87
Brooten, Dorothy, 190
Businessmen, vs. businesswomen, 100t

Career roles. See Leadership; Nursing.
Caring, and excellence, 184
CCNE (Commission on Collegiate Nursing Education), 148

Central Virginia Nursing Leadership Institute, 162
Chaleff, I., 54–55
Change, 10, 122, 127–128
agents of, 123–125, 188
barriers to, 128
behavior of healthcare executives during, 126t
conflict generated by, 128–129
facilitation of, 125–126
life impulses and, 86
moving phase of, 127
principles of, 123
process of, 127–128
readiness for, quantification of, 126, 131f–133f
refreezing phase of, 127
"ripple effect" of, 141
unfreezing phase of, 127
Change agents, 123–125, 188
Chaos, 25, 117–119
leadership in presence of, 121–122
nursing and, 119–120
Chaos theory, 25–27
Chapman University, 158
Choreography, in balancing demands, 184
Christ, Jesus, 47
Chrysler, 84

Coaching, 124
Coercive power, 47
Cognitive development, 29
Collaboration, 138
Comfort, with conflict, 189
Co-missioning, 25, 71
Commission on Collegiate
    Nursing Education (CCNE),
    148
Communication, by leaders, 9
    by nurses, 9–10
    of vision, 84
Competence, 62
    and credibility, 46
Complexity theory, 30
Computers, data display
    capability of, 25
Conflict, avoidance of, 129
    change and, 128–129
    comfort with, 189
    management of, case study of,
    129–130
Confusion, 31
Continuity, 10
Contributor style, of followership,
    43
Cost(s), of healthcare, 143
    containment of, 115
    prediction of, 143
Courage, 25
Course work, 158
"Crafty" leaders, 90
Creativity, 85–90
    case study of, in developing
    vision, 88
    mindmap of, 87f
    tool for assessing, 90, 94–96
Credibility, of leaders, 46, 68–69
Crichton, Michael, 118–119
Critical pathways, 76
Critical reflection, and excellence,
    183

Data display capability, of com-
    puters, 25
Delivery systems, integrated, 145
Demographic trends, 143. See also
    Future trends.
Dependent/independent
    parameters, of followership,
    42f
Diamond model, of leadership, 83
Discipline, and excellence, 184

Discussions, participation in, 158
Disequilibrium, 29, 30
Dissonance, 30
Distance education, for nurses,
    146
Dreher, Melanie, 190

Education, and leadership,
    158–162
    and nursing, 146, 148
    excellence in, 187
Effective followers, 41, 44–46
Elderly patients, healthcare needs
    of, 143
Emotional intelligence, 65–66
    case study of, 65
Empowerment, 48–49, 167–168
Energy, positive vs. negative
    contributors to, 27
Erikson, Erik, 30
Esteem, 66–67
Evans, Lois, 190
Excellence, 181–191
    academic, 187
    caring and, 184
    critical reflection and, 183
    discipline and, 184
    indifference to, case study of,
    182
    leadership in relation to, 187,
    189
    nursing in relation to, 186
    passion and, 184
    perseverance and, 184
    responsibility and, 184
    skepticism and, 184
    striving for, 183
    case study of, 182
Executive wisdom, 124
Exemplary followers, 41, 44–46
Expert power, 47
Explaining, 4, 48

"Feisty" leaders, 90
Fellowship(s), leadership educa-
    tion provided by, 161–162
"Femaleness," 100
    combining "maleness" with, 106
Five-P model, of followers, 43–44
Florida Atlantic University, 161
Focus, and leadership, 116–117
    vs. focus in management, 6t
    in typology of vision, 76, 77f

Follower(s), 41–44. See also
    Followership.
    alienated, 41
    case study of, 41
    development of, 11–13
    effective/exemplary, 41, 44–46
    five-P model of, 43–44
    leaders in relation to, 11–13,
    36, 38, 44t. See also
    Leader(s).
    conceptualizations of, 37f
    motivation of, 48
    recognition of importance
    of, 3
    sheep label applied to, 42
    types of, 41–44, 42f
    working with, 125t
    yes-people, 41–42
Followership, 36, 39–40, 43f.
    See also Follower(s).
    contributor style of, 43
    development of, 49–53
    independent/dependent
    parameters of, 42f
    partner style of, 43
    passive/active parameters of,
    42f
    politician style of, 43
    subordinate style of, 43
    tool for assessing, 56–57
"Footprints" (Bagley), 92
Ford, Henry, 8
Fort Hays State University, 158
Freedom-related differences,
    between leadership and
    management, 6t
Full-time equivalent RNs, 146
Futurescan, 139
Future trends, 142–143
    in healthcare, 143–145, 145t
    in nursing, 145–151
    leadership characteristics
    and, 151–153
Futurists, 139

Gandhi, Mahatma, 8
Gardner, John, 185
Gates, Bill, 78
Geese, 70
Gender perspectives, in
    leadership, 99–111
    androgynous approaches
    and, 106, 107t

businessman/businesswoman
roles and, 100t
case study of, 108
"femaleness" and, 100, 106
"maleness" and, 100, 106
mentoring and, 170
stereotyping and, 99
strategies for success and,
108–110
Geriatric patients, healthcare
needs of, 143
Goal(s), 4, 5
vs. vision, 76. *See also* Vision.
Goal-related differences,
between leadership and
management, 6t
Great Man theory, of leadership,
2, 157
Grossman-Valiga leadership
assessment tool, 16–19
Group representation, 4
Guides, 173

Havel, Vaclev, 50
Healthcare. *See also* Nursing;
Patient(s).
aging population's needs for,
143
costs of, 143
containment of, 115
prediction of, 143
future of, 143–145, 145t
improvement of, 140
promotion of, 187
inpatient, 142
quality of, 144
registered nurse's role in,
120–121
traditional systems of, 145t
Healthcare executives,
behavior of, during
change, 126t
Helene Fuld Health Trust, 162
Henderson, Virginia, 190
Heroes, 50
Honesty, and credibility, 46
Honor Society of Nursing, 161
"How Creative Are You?", 90,
94–96
Humility, 25

"I Have A Dream," 79
Iacocca, Lee, 84

IDSs (integrated delivery
systems), 145
If (Kipling), 14–15
IHI (Institute for Healthcare
Improvement), 187
Independent/dependent
parameters, of followership,
42f
Industrial age, movement away
from, 28
INHL (Institute for Nursing
Healthcare Leadership), 161
INL (Institute for Nursing
Leadership), 161
Innovation-related differences,
between leadership and
management, 6t
Inpatient healthcare, 142
Inspiration, and credibility, 46.
See also Vision.
Institute(s), leadership education
provided by, 161–162
Institute for Healthcare
Improvement (IHI), 187
Institute for Nursing Healthcare
Leadership (INHL), 161
Institute for Nursing Leadership
(INL), 161
Integrated delivery systems
(IDSs), 145
Integrative function, of leaders,
137–138
Intelligence, emotional, 65–66
case study of, 65
International Center for Health
Leadership, 162
IQ (intelligence quotient),
vs. emotional intelligence, 65

Jesus Christ, 47
Job training, 162
Jobs, Steve, 8

Kennesaw State University, 158
King, Imogene, 190
King, Martin Luther, Jr., 8, 79
Kipling, Rudyard, 14–15

Leader(s). *See also* Leadership.
change agent, 123–125, 188
collaboration fostered by, 138
communication by, 9
"crafty," 90

credibility of, 46, 68–69
"feisty," 90
followers in relation to, 11–13,
36, 38, 44t. *See also*
Follower(s).
conceptualizations of, 37f
integrative function of,
137–138
women as, 101, 102–106. *See
also* Leadership, gender
perspectives in.
strategies for, 108–110
would-be, 67–68
Leadership, 7–13. *See also*
Leader(s).
adjusting to, 116–117
alpha, 102
androgynous, 106, 107t.
See also Leadership,
gender perspectives in.
beta, 102
contemporary theories of, 3
development/facilitation of,
24–25, 158–164
case study of, 164
environments for,
165–168
assessment of, 166t
in presence of chaos,
121–122
diamond model of, 83
education and, 158–162
elements of, 7–13
excellence in relation to, 187,
189
gender perspectives in, 99–111
androgynous approaches
and, 106, 107t
businessman/businesswoman
roles and, 100t
case study of, 108
"femaleness" and, 100, 106
"maleness" and, 100, 106
mentoring and, 170
stereotyping and, 99
strategies for success and,
108–110
Great Man theory of, 2, 157
legendary, 81
new science of, 29
case study of, 29
nursing, 24–25, 62–69. *See also*
Nursing.

futurist perspective on,
151–153
participative focus and,
116–117
personal trait theories of, 2
principle-centered, 68
situational theories of, 2–3
tasks of, 4
theories of, 2–3
tools for assessing, 16–20, 166t
trait theories of, 2
transactional, 63
transformational, 63–65
types of, 63–65
vision in relation to, 7–9, 46,
64, 188. *See also* Vision.
vs. management, 4–7, 6t
Leadership image, 66–67
Leadership Initiative for Nursing
Education (LINE), 162
Lectures, participation in, 158
Left-sided brain functions, 87
Legendary leadership, 81
Legitimate power, 47
Life/change dynamic, 86
Lightner, Candy, 8, 188
LINE (Leadership Initiative for
Nursing Education), 162
Lombardi, Vince, 185

MADD (Mothers Against Drunk
Driving), 188
"Maleness," 100
combining "femaleness" with,
106
Management, 4–7, 6t. *See also*
Leadership.
Maslow, A., 66
"Meditation on Followership,"
55
Mentoring, 12, 168–172, 171t
myths about, 169–170
Mother Teresa, 8, 78
Mothers Against Drunk Driving
(MADD), 188
Motivation, 4, 48
Moving phase, of change, 127

National League of Nursing
Accrediting Commission
(NLNAC), 148
National Student Nurses
Association (NSNA), 159

Negative energy, persons creating,
27
Networking, 172–173
myths about, 173t
New science, 26, 27–29
of leadership, case study of, 29
Newtonian age, movement away
from, 28
Nightingale, Florence, 8
NLI (Nursing Leadership
Institute), 161
NLNAC (National League of
Nursing Accrediting
Commission), 148
NSNA (National Student Nurses
Association), 159
Nurse(s), 61. *See also* Nursing
entries.
case study of input by, in practice setting, 152–153
communication by, 9–10
registered, 29, 120–121
full-time equivalent, 146
positions for, 142, 146
Nursing. *See also* Nurse(s);
Healthcare.
accreditation bodies in, recommendations of, 148
chaos in, 119–120
education and, 146, 148
excellence in, 186
future of, 145–151
leadership and, 151–153
institutional facilitation of, 161,
162
leadership and, 24–25, 62–69.
See also Leadership.
futurist perspective on,
151–153
relationship-based model of,
64
Nursing Leadership Institute
(NLI), 161

Occupational training, 162
Older patients, healthcare needs
of, 143
On-the-job training, 162
Order-related differences,
between leadership and
management, 6t
Organizational readiness-to-change
quotient, 132f

Orientation, in typology of
vision, 76, 77f

Participative focus, and leader-
ship, 116–117
Partner style, of followership,
42–43
Partnering, 150–151
Passion, and excellence, 184
Passive/active parameters, of
followership, 42f
Pathways, critical, 76
Patient(s). *See also* Healthcare.
coordination between primary
care provider and, 120
emotionally intelligent care of,
case study of, 65
in-hospital care of, 142
older, healthcare needs of, 143
Patient outcomes, 146
Peer "pals," 173
Performance initiatives, 42
Perseverance, and excellence, 184
Personal attention, 12
Personal trait theories, of
leadership, 2
Personal vision, 77
Personnel mix, 26
Perspective transformation,
30–31
Perspective-related differences,
between leadership and
management, 6t
Pesut, Dan, 190
Phi Kappa Phi, 189, 190
Pioneer Leadership Program, 159
Pittman, Robert, 8
Plausible future, 140. *See also*
Future trends.
Politician style, of followership,
43
Population trends, 143. *See also*
Future trends.
Position-related differences,
between leadership and
management, 6t
Positive energy, persons creating,
27
Possibilities, vs. adversities, 118
Possible future, 140. *See also*
Future trends.
Power, 46–47, 167
Power Perception Profile, 47

Power-base differences,
  between leadership and
  management, 6t
The Power Tactics of Jesus Christ, 47
Precepting, 12
Preferred future, 140. *See also*
  Future trends.
Primary care provider, coordina-
  tion between patient and,
  120
Principle-centered leadership, 68
Probable future, 140. *See also*
  Future trends.
Professional roles. See Leadership;
  Nursing.
Professional vision, 77
Protégés, mentors and, 170,
  171t

Quality, 144, 184. *See also*
  Excellence.
Quantum theory, 27–29
"Queen Bee syndrome," 101

Readiness-to-change quotient,
  126, 131f–133f
Reconceptualization, 31
Referent power, 47
Reflection, 163
  critical, and excellence, 183
Refreezing phase, of change, 127
Registered nurses (RNs), 29,
  120–121
  full-time equivalent, 146
  positions for, 142, 146
Relationship(s), 5
Relationship-Based Nursing Model,
  64–15
Relationship initiatives, 42
Renewal, 4, 11–12, 48
Resolution, 31
Responsibility, and excellence,
  184
Reward power, 47
Right-sided brain functions, 87
"Ripple effect," of change, 141
Risk-level differences,
  between leadership and
  management, 6t
RNs (registered nurses), 29,
  120–121
  full-time equivalent, 146
  positions for, 142, 146

Role modeling, 12, 160–161
Role-playing, 159–160

Saturation, 31
Science (new science), 26, 27–29
  of leadership, case study of, 29
Self, sense of, 5–6
Self-actualization, 66
Self-assessment, 163
Self-assessment tool, for creativity,
  90, 94–96
  for followership style, 56–57
  for leadership skills, 20
  for readiness to change, 131f
Self-esteem, 66–67
Self-organizing systems, 27, 89
Sensitivity training, 160
Sexual stereotyping, 99
Sheep label, as applied to
  followers, 42
Sigma Theta Tau, 161, 182, 189,
  190
Simulation, 159–160
Situational theories, of leader-
  ship, 2–3
Skepticism, and excellence, 184
Smith, Fred, 8
SNA (Student Nurses
  Association), 159
Sponsors, 173
Stability, 30
  return to, 31
Staff mix, 26
Stereotyping, gender-based, 99
Stewardship, 11
Strumpf, Neville, 190
Student Nurses Association
  (SNA), 159
Subordinate style, of follower-
  ship, 43
Symbol, individual(s) serving as,
  4, 48
Synthesis, 31

Task completion, transactional
  leadership and, 63
Team(s), 125t
Thinking, whole-brain, 87
Traditional healthcare systems,
  145t
Training, on-the-job, 162
  sensitivity, 160
Trait theories, of leadership, 2

Transactional leadership, 63
Transformation, perspective,
  30–31
Transformational leadership,
  63–65

Uncertainty, dealing with, 31
Unfreezing phase, of change, 127
Unity, workable, 4, 48
University of Denver, 159
University of Illinois at Chicago,
  162
University of Richmond, 158

Values, affirmation of, 4, 48
Vision, 76–85
  absence of, effects of, 81
  actualization of, 78–81
  communication of, 84
  creativity and, 88
    case study of, 88
  credibility in relation to, 46
  development of, 81–83
    case study of, 88
  leadership and, 7–9, 46, 64,
    188. *See also* Leadership.
  personal, 77
  professional, 77
  typology of, 77f
    focus in, 76, 77f
    orientation in, 76, 77f
  vs. goals, 76
Vision-related differences,
  between leadership and management, 6t

Walton, Sam, 8
West Virginia Nursing Leadership
  Institute, 162
Whole-brain thinking, 87
Wisdom, executive, 124
Women, as leaders, 101, 102–106.
  See also Leadership, gender
  perspectives in.
  strategies for, 108–110
Work, conceptions of, 5
Workable unity, 4, 48
Workplace training, 162

Yes people, 41–42